DIZZY

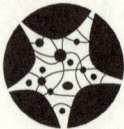

CONNECTIVE TISSUE

A Health Humanities and Narrative Medicine Series
Renée K. Nicholson, Series Editor

CONNECTIVE TISSUE is a series in health humanities and narrative medicine that illuminates lived experiences with health, illness, and medicine. This series explores innovative approaches to healthcare by integrating expressive arts and humanities practices into therapeutic settings and generating works of creative writing that artfully render stories of illness, disability, and the journey to well-being.

Dizzy: A Memoir
Rachel Weaver

DIZZY

a memoir

Rachel Weaver

West Virginia University Press | Morgantown

First edition published 2026 by West Virginia University Press

Printed in the United States of America

ISBN 978-1-959000-74-7 (paperback)/ISBN 978-1-959000-75-4 (ePub) /
ISBN 978-1-959000-84-6 (PDF)

Library of Congress Cataloging-in-Publication Data

Names: Weaver, Rachel, 1974- author

Title: Dizzy : a memoir / Rachel Weaver.

Description: First edition. | Morgantown : West Virginia University
Press, 2026. | Series: Connective tissue ; 1 Identifiers:
LCCN 2025032652 | ISBN 9781959000747 paperback |
ISBN 9781959000754 ebook

Subjects: LCSH: Weaver, Rachel, 1974– | Weaver, Rachel, 1974—Health |
Authors, American—21st century—Biography | Women authors,
American—Biography | Dizziness—Patients | LCGFT: Autobiographies

Classification: LCC PS3623.E386 Z46 2026

LC record available at https://lccn.loc.gov/2025032652

Cover design by Michel Vrana

Book design by Ashley Muehlbauer / AM Book Design

Cover painting by Alex Garant

For EU safety/GPSR concerns, please direct inquiries to WVUPress@
mail.wvu.edu or our physical mailing address at West Virginia
University Press / PO Box 6295 / West Virginia University /
Morgantown, WV, 26508, USA.

For anyone lost in the dark.
Me too, for so long.

ACKNOWLEDGMENTS

Some material in this book originally appeared in *The Sun Magazine*, *River Teeth*, *Southeast Review*, *Tulip Tree Review*, *Medicine and Meaning*, *New Letters Magazine*, the *North American Review*, and in the anthology *We Can See Into Another Place* (Bower House, 2024). I am grateful to these publications for first bringing the work to light.

Thanks to Dr. Tanner for making room in his care to address the mental hardship of chronic illness as well as the physical. The two together were driving me toward a specific end, and his effort to make room for both in our weekly appointments made all the difference.

Without Dr. Bills's innovative approach to migraine science, I'd still be stuck in jail. Not sure how to say thank you for that. There really aren't words.

I'd also like to thank my agent, Andrea Somberg, who has been such a strong supporter of this project. Thanks to Renée Nicholson and Marguerite Avery at WVU Press for believing in this book as well.

Mike, Nate, and Wes—the three of you have always made room for my health struggle and loved me through all of it. Despite periodically posting the No Boys Allowed sign outside my writing shed, I don't really mean it.

AUTHOR'S NOTE

Throughout all of the events depicted in this narrative, I was severely compromised in both the way my mind was working and how physically uncomfortable I was. I have done my best to recall accurately what happened, but there are likely minor missteps, for which I take full responsibility. In a few cases, I've combined two separate events into one for narrative clarity. Some names have been changed to protect those individuals' privacy.

DIZZY

BEFORE

It was the moonlight that made me forget to pay attention. The way the sky opened up over the forgotten parts of Alaska after forty days of thirty-five degrees and rain. The temperature fell for a week straight, and the river outside of town froze solid. Or solid enough.

I laced up my cold skates, the freedom of the ice already buzzing in my chest. I scooted across the rocks to the edge of the wide, frozen river, scooted out a little further, and stood up. There is a point of balance on skates, elusive but there, always there. My body adjusted, found it, and settled in. I pushed off, my skates gliding through the imperfections in the ice, legs absorbing the bump and rattle of the way it froze.

I weighted my foot and took off at a sprint, upstream, into the wind, into the night. Underfoot, there and then gone, a salmon frozen in the ice, belly up, spawned out.

With every solid push off my inside edge, the difficulties of no money, an angry boyfriend, the lack of a plan for my life cleaved off in huge chunks. There was only the pull of my lungs against the cold night, the sound of something big and wild moving up ahead along the shoreline, thousands of feet of rocks and trees on either side, glowing. The natural world always made sense in a way people did not. It was the only thing I felt deeply connected to.

And then the quick crack, the ice opening, my shins exploding in pain, the icy water filling my thick work pants, stealing the scream from my chest.

YEAR ONE

CHAPTER ONE

January 2006.

On the day that would become the line between Before and After, I opened my eyes to the walls of the bedroom folding and sliding and picking up speed. In the dim, blue-gray light of morning, the room gathered itself into a proper hurricane. I squeezed my eyes shut. I'd felt fine when I'd gone to bed the previous night. I had not been drinking. Nothing like this had ever happened before. With my eyes closed, I was flung weightless and spinning through dark space.

I opened my eyes wide and pressed my body hard against the mattress in search of the center, the still place. Anyplace. My hands frantic for something firm to hold onto, but everything was moving with me. Karl, my boyfriend, still asleep next to me on the bed that had been picked up by the angry arms of the hurricane, rolled just out of reach when I grasped for him.

Desperate to get away from whatever was happening, I pushed the covers off inch by inch, keeping my head as still as possible, and slid down to all fours next to the bed. I set my sights on the hallway. I was clawing more than crawling, the carpet rushing beneath my hands like a river just let loose from a dam.

In the hallway, panting, I slowly got my feet under me, crouched low, hands spidered against the carpet. I pressed my shoulder up against the wall so I knew where it was and slowly stood. I made it to the bathroom by slithering along the wall. If I could just brush my teeth, maybe have some coffee, I figured things would right themselves.

I stood in the bathroom, took four slow deep breaths, forcing the rest of the sleep from my head, and the spinning slowed. I bent slowly and splashed water onto my face. Wiped it mostly dry with a hand and peered at myself in the mirror. Maybe this was a panic attack.

Seven days earlier, I had packed up a life I loved in Alaska to start a two year creative writing graduate program in Colorado. Karl had come along to help with the move. That particular morning, he would begin the 2,500 mile trek back home without me. Somewhere in the swirling distance, I heard his alarm go off. We were staying with a friend of mine I'd met on a boat years before. I'd be there until I moved into the house of a single mom I didn't know and her four kids. I had just paid off my undergraduate loans and was determined to squeak by somehow without borrowing money for graduate school. The single mom needed someone to make dinners four nights a week and had an empty basement she was willing to offer up as a trade. I didn't know how to cook or what kids ate but was going to figure it out in order to live in a basement for free. I also needed a full-time job or two that I could work around a full class schedule. The ill-fated plan was to finish school and get back to the perfect little A-frame cabin on the water, tucked between hemlock and spruce, always fogged in just enough to remind you winter was coming.

In the brightly colored, cheery bathroom, I took a deep breath. Breathing helped with panic attacks, I'd heard. The hurricane had subsided, but the bathroom sloshed and rolled as if I were out in the Bering Sea, clinging to a life raft. The walls shimmied in my vision like thin curtains in a breeze. I rubbed my eyes, splayed my hands out on the counter, and told myself it was solid and still. I just had to wait it out. I was good at waiting things out.

Karl shot me a steely look as he stepped past me to the toilet and peed hard enough to peel paint. We'd fought the night before. Over the past few months, he'd made sure to let me know exactly what he thought as I tossed away the life we scrabbled to build: the handful of trusted friends, all the winter wood cut and stacked, the freezer full of halibut, salmon, and crab we'd caught. All to pursue a tugging dream of my own, separate from him.

I thought about telling him what was happening, but meeting his eyes felt like aggression, and words like too much. Instead, I concentrated on getting the toothpaste on the toothbrush as he stepped into the shower.

I pulled on jeans and a sweatshirt back in the bedroom, moving in slow motion, afraid I'd set the room to spinning again if I moved my head at all. Maybe I just needed to sleep. There hadn't been much of that in the past week. Pavement and buildings and people made me feel hemmed in, anxious. And everything was so loud and constant. I wanted to be surrounded by slow moving water, light, cool wind, and woods full of bears. But bigger than that was this dream of writing books.

The entire bedroom tilted quickly to the left. I reached out and caught the bed that was, without warning, above me, about to crash down. Breathless and gasping, crumpled on the floor, my heart pounded as my brain forced the walls back where they should be, assured me that the bed had not just been hovering over me.

A cold sweat broke out across my forehead. Whatever the problem was, I decided, I could will it away. I stood up straight, concentrated on a corner of the room. *This still wall meets that still wall meets that still carpet,* I told myself. The walls shimmered again in a breeze and then stilled as if blown out. The carpet river widened and slowed. I breathed in and out, focused on the fact that I had control. And then the wind picked up, and the river banked, and the walls and floor slid out from under me.

Karl bustled into the room. "We're going to be late," he said, gathering his strewn about clothes and shoving them in his worn out brown duffel. I watched his hands. Thought about everything they could fix. "The ticket cost a fortune. I don't want to miss the bus."

I didn't say anything. It was always best to just let him do what he needed to do. I only sort of knew what set him off, and I never knew what calmed him down. I did know that I couldn't possibly handle one extra thing that morning. I slid my feet into Xtratufs, the rubber boot uniform of southeast Alaska and the only footwear I owned. Appropriate for the rainy winters of coastal Alaska, as well as the rainy rest of the year of coastal Alaska, but thin and not warm enough for Colorado winter.

Coffee sounded terrible as I made my way down the stairs in the early morning light. Karl didn't drink coffee, and even though

I thought caffeine might right things, I knew it was going to be easier if I didn't hold him up by making myself some. I grabbed a bagel off the kitchen counter, checked that my keys were still in my jeans pocket, and followed him out the door.

Karl drove us to the bus station in morning interstate traffic while I sat gripping the seat with one hand, the other splayed out against the passenger door, every muscle tensed.

"Are you okay?" he asked, glancing over. His shoulder length, dark hair was tied back in a low, smooth ponytail. His glasses were cleaner than I'd ever seen them. Usually, his hair was frizzed out, gathering the misty light rain, his glasses streaked with it. Usually, we were in a skiff fishing, or bushwhacking through the rainforest with heavy packs. He looked weird in traffic, untouched by weather.

"Yeah," I said, staring at the car's taillights ahead of us. "I don't know what it is. It'll pass. I feel seasick. I think."

He threw me a surprised look. I was the one who could stay out in all weather, who loved to fly with Noel, the Vietnam-flashback bush pilot everyone else dreaded climbing into a plane with, the one who could carry on full conversations in a helicopter circling endlessly to locate the exact location of a goshawk nest we would hike in so we could check the number of young they'd managed that year.

But on a straight highway across the plains, I felt as if I were on a roller coaster after having shotgunned multiple beers. I checked the shoulder of the highway, considered asking him to pull over, to take me home. He'd miss his bus. Or maybe he could just pull over and I could walk the miles back and then curl up and sleep until everything stilled. Karl could leave my car at the bus terminal, and I would figure out how to get it back later.

I did none of this.

I set my teeth through the rest of the car trip, followed Karl into the bus station, and sat on a hard plastic chair while he checked in.

"Well," he said, sitting back down, paper ticket in hand. "See you this summer, I guess?" His face cracked then, and I saw through the frustration to the hurt. We'd been together several years, wanted the same thing out of life: to live outside the typical expectations. We loved the same things: cold seas, untouched land, and the unpredictability of wild animals. We'd slowly accumulated crab pots, commercial halibut gear, old kayaks; we'd rebuilt an old wooden skiff, had paddled and explored together until the wild places felt like home.

"Yeah," I said. The plan with all the holes in it was that he would spend the summer in Colorado or I would spend the summer in Alaska. We both preferred that I go back to Alaska, but I had a month-long course to complete in the middle of the summer, and he didn't want to be in Colorado.

When his bus pulled up, he wrapped his arms around me. Against his familiar chest for half a second, I relaxed. He scooped his duffel off the floor next to us, threw it over his shoulder, pushed through the door out to the bus lanes, and got in line. I slumped back into the hard chair and watched all the familiar angles of him through the grimy glass as he disappeared into the bus.

The overwaxed orange tile floor pulled loose and sloshed around as I tried to figure out how I was going to drive home. Fear spiraled up through me like a thick snake, and I felt sure I was going to throw up.

The bus hissed and pulled out; a plastic grocery bag tossed in its wake. I needed to drive back, I needed to find a job, I needed to go to orientation for grad school later that day. I got to my feet, which felt far away and not really a part of me. An invisible force pulled me hard left. I fought it, leaning hard right, and angled for the door. In a cloud of nerves, nausea, and fear, I found my car on a side street, unlocked it, and slid into the driver's seat.

I pulled out of the parking spot before I had enough time to chicken out. If I closed one eye, the lines painted on the road moved less. I felt disconnected to my hands on the wheel, to the thoughts in my mind. It was as if the conscious part of me had been pulled and stretched apart from the physical part. We were still tethered, but the line was threading.

The oncoming cars jumped and swerved slightly in my vision, so I hugged the right side, looping wide around bikers in too tight clothes. It occurred to me that I should pull over, but then what? Who to call? There was no one. I merged onto the highway.

I white-knuckled, one-eyed it back up the interstate and drove straight to the student health center on campus. I had two hours before orientation. Once parked, I slumped over the steering wheel. The car continued to lurch and swing underneath me. I pressed my chest harder against the steering wheel, trying to attach myself to the heavy stillness of the car. Terror vined through me, prickling my neck in the way it always did, except this was worse than a Cessna ride through fogged-in mountaintops, worse than the locked gaze of a pissed-off brown bear. I looked up at the health center across the street, unsure I could even make it up the stairs and inside.

■ ■ ■

"Help you?" the woman at the reception desk said. I held onto the edge of the desk, planted my feet wide to keep from falling over.

"I need to see a doctor."

"What's the issue?"

"I'm dizzy."

She made a noncommittal noise and turned to her computer. She asked my name and address. She flicked her gaze up when I recited my PO box in Alaska. The lady with the four kids lived on a crowded street, but I didn't know the name of it. "Insurance card?"

"I bought the university health insurance."

"Oh," she said. "Are you a new student?"

"Yes."

"Well, the plan doesn't actually take effect until the semester starts, which is still five days away."

I watched her mouth move and tried to understand what she was saying. It was as though she were leaning over a tub of water that I was submerged in. *Five days*, I heard, *five days*. I would not survive another five days of this. *Out of pocket*, she said in the watery distance. Yes, I nodded, yes. The money would run out soon, but surely I had enough to pay for one doctor's visit? The job search was to start next. I tried to imagine going to an interview in my current state. I needed a medical professional to treat it, to stop it, so that I could find a job, start school, and manage the weird living situation I'd arranged for myself. All of these things needed to happen immediately. I handed over my credit card.

The numbers jumped and slid off the receipt. $120, I made out. *Okay, alright,* I thought, *that's not too bad.* The signature line was a snaky slither, impossible to pin down. The last half of my last name ended up scribbled on the desk.

I leaned heavily into the wall to stay upright as I was ushered back to an exam room. Ten minutes later, a momish nurse practitioner bustled into the room. She settled the soft roundness of herself on the stool and fixed me with a worried look as I clung to the exam table and tried not to move a single part of my body.

"What can I do for you today?" Her voice was smooth like balm.

"Woke up dizzy," I said, keeping my eyes fixed on a black smear on the floor, a complete sentence beyond me.

"Any other symptoms?" She rolled an inch closer. Maybe I looked as though I were about to topple over? Maybe I was toppling over?

"No," I muttered.

"Anything happen that might've caused this? A hit to the head? A car accident?" She put one hand on my knee. The touch almost made me cry with relief. She would help.

"No."

Her brows furrowed. "Anything significant in your medical history?"

"No. Nothing like this has ever happened before."

She placed cold hands on my back and chest as she listened to my heart, poked around in my ears, and shone a pinprick of light in my eyes. She sat back on the rolly chair and gently laid her hand on my knee again, as if trying to help still me. Her dark eyes were clouded with worry.

"Have you gone through any major life changes recently?"

"I left a lot behind to start graduate school."

"Did you want to leave?"

I winced. The physical pain of the question caught me off guard.

"Hmm," she said, slow and thoughtful. "This could just be too much stress," she concluded.

Three months earlier, I had been trapped in the elbow of a slow moving river by a five-hundred-pound brown bear and her three cubs, the banks on either side too steep for me or her to climb. I had spent forty-five minutes keeping the mother bear in the sight of my rifle—finger on the trigger, safety off—as she snapped her jaws, paced, and false charged twice. Not even a tinge of dizziness that day.

"Pretty sure it's not just stress," I said.

She tilted her head a little, considering. "Your ears have a lot of wax in them. Maybe cleaning them out will help."

She ushered me into another, smaller room, where a boy not old enough to order a whiskey squirted a hard stream of water into my ear. The room pitched left, the sink lifted over my head and then swung behind me. I gripped the plastic chair beneath me, trying to find a still center. The boy squirted another hard blast of water, and everything around me pulled free and whipped up into a wild spin, worse than the hurricane I'd woken up to.

I made some sort of guttural sound, swung an arm out, caught him in the chest, and rolled out of the plastic chair onto the cold linoleum floor. On my hands and knees, I tried to merge myself into what I knew was still. But the room continued to spin at a furious speed. Shoes raced past me as I spread-eagled and tried to dig my fingernails into the floor. The nurse practitioner's hands were on my back, trying to coax me off the floor. But to sit up was to not know where the floor was. I had to know where the floor was to know where I was. I pressed my cheek hard against the dirty linoleum.

From some great watery distance, she said, "I'm going to get you in to see the ENT right now." She reappeared with a pillow as the hurricane was blowing itself out. "Can we get you off the floor?" She wrapped an arm around my waist and guided me into the nearest exam room. On the hard plastic, I curled into the smallest ball I could make of myself. "The ENT office is across town. Is there someone I can call?" she asked, her hand making small circles on my back. My brother was in Texas, my mom in Michigan, my friend who I was staying with was an elementary school teacher and was at work. I had an aunt and uncle in town, but my aunt had slept with some dude who tie-dyed socks, and they were in the midst of a horrible divorce.

"I'll be okay," I whispered, eyes fixed on the sharp corner of the counter. "If I can just lay here for a bit."

■ ■ ■

Forty-five minutes later, I was back in the driver's seat, the spinning back to a sloshing, my whole body buzzing with what ifs. What if this lasted all week? What if I missed the beginning of classes? What if it was a brain tumor? What if I couldn't handle it?

I closed one eye and backed out of the parking space.

■ ■ ■

"Insurance card?" the receptionist asked me in a bright, airy, windowed front room of the ENT's office.

I held tight to the edge of the desk with both hands. "I bought the university insurance, but apparently it doesn't start until next Monday."

"No supplemental insurance?" Her mascara was thick and precise, every lash attended to. She smelled of fake fruity lotion, which made bile claw up my throat.

"Just catastrophic," I said.

"Well, that won't help." She gave me a look like I should start contributing to society. "Out of pocket is $350." Which was more than I'd spent in the past month combined and more than half what I currently had. I'd been so careful with money, knowing it had to stretch to cover the transition from leaving one job and finding another.

Chasing your dreams is all well and good. Another good one: money matters less than happiness. I dreamed up a life full of adventure and that made me happy. I loved loading up in helicopters for a day of work, getting dropped off with an aerial photo and a compass on an uninhabited island full of bears in terrible weather, and that tingly, alive feeling produced by the fact that any kind of shit might go down at any moment and probably would. But adventure only paid $13,000 a year, which meant scrambling for winter work wherever I could find it in a town that mostly shut down in the winter. It meant hours spent catching halibut, salmon, and crab to fill the freezer because I couldn't afford meat at the grocery store.

I fought against the tears that were suddenly rising, along with some prickly new sense of shame in this city where the proper thing to do was fill a freezer with meat from Costco, drive to work, and pad your 401(k).

I handed over my credit card.

The ENT was in a hurry. He whipped into the room, white coattails fluttering in a way that set the room to sloshing. He glanced over at me gripping the armrests of the chair in the middle of the room that was reclined just enough to suggest submission. "Okay," he said as he settled on the rolly stool and jiggled the mouse to wake up the computer. The time flashed on the screen, and I vaguely registered that orientation had started without me.

I wanted to tell him that I was missing it, that I'd just watched my boyfriend walk away, that my body had never done anything like this to me before. That it had always been strong and resilient, something to trust, sometimes the only thing to trust. That I was more tired than I ever thought possible. That life in the rain is hard.

"Looks like you didn't fill out the paperwork in the waiting room," he said, clearly annoyed.

The words and lines had swum around on the page. I'd had to close my eyes and focus on not puking on the patterned carpet. It hadn't seemed worth blowing chunks to fill in a bunch of blanks about the three drunk grandparents I'd barely known and the one I had known who was addicted to pills. I didn't know anything about high blood pressures or heart conditions for any of them. What I did know a lot about was the generational fallout of four people's poor choices.

"I tried—" I started, but he interrupted.

"We'll just have to do it now," he said with a do-I-have-to-do-everything sigh.

I did my best to answer his monotony of questions about the health concerns of people not in the room, of the surgery on my elbow at age ten, using up all the energy I was hoping to spend on discussing loose walls and river floors. He intently watched the screen, engaged in the difficult task of entering the year of my elbow surgery in the correct narrow field. After all the history questions, he asked the screen of the computer, "So, you're dizzy. Any other symptoms?"

"No," I said. "It's—" *Pretty bad*, I wanted to explain, but he spun around so quickly, I had to close my eyes to keep the spinning from continuing from him to the edges of the room. He was focused on snapping an endpiece on his ear probe and didn't ask me to finish, so I dropped it. He probed around for a bit and then sat back on his stool. "Lot of wax in there." He popped the endpiece into the trash and turned back to his computer. "I'm referring you to a physical therapist who specializes in the vestibular system, which controls balance and stabilizes eye movements. Can't get you in until tomorrow. Nancy at the front desk will give you all the necessary info." And then he was bustling out in the same way he'd bustled in ten minutes previous.

For thirty-five dollars a minute, he'd learned a lot about my relatives and nothing about me.

■ ■ ■

The following day, I lay on crinkly paper with my head in a stranger's hands. I'd slept the entire afternoon the day before and missed all of orientation.

The physical therapist was a friendly, bubbly woman. She was talking so fast, I had to squint through the fog in my brain to keep up. "Benign positional vertigo," she was saying behind me, the firm pads of her fingers searching either side of my head for the best grip. *Benign*, I thought, latching onto the word like a life ring: not harmful, gentle even. *Benign,* I said again to myself.

The bright Colorado sun was burning across the room in sharp, vertical slashes. I missed the way the cool misty mornings of southeast Alaska left you alone. The vertical slashes became wild streaks of light as they spun in my vision. I wanted to close the blinds tight, but the physical therapist had a firm grip on my head.

As her fingers found purchase, my whole body tensed. I had no idea what she was going to do. I only knew it was imperative that my head remain still or the room would turn into a hurricane that could last for hours. Maybe days. I tried to interrupt her monologue about benign positional vertigo as her fingers stretched further across my skull, perhaps anticipating the fight.

"Basically, you have a basket of crystals in your inner ear," she was explaining. "Those crystals need to stay in the basket, but every once in a while, one will fall out. What we need to do is a series of quick motions with your head to get that crystal to fall back into the basket."

"No," I said. I did not want my head moved at all, much less quickly. But I was a scientist, and this was science. It made sense, sort of, the basket and the crystals. And with the desperation of someone lost at sea, I wanted more than anything to get back to shore.

"Okay," I said, my whole body pulsing with a hot, sweaty fear as her fingers tightened around my skull.

She whipped my head to the right and then sharply left, had me roll onto my side for ninety seconds and then sit up quickly. Silent tears burned down my cheeks, and my heart pounded in my throat as the bright stripes of sun whipped past like cars swerving wildly at night. I white-knuckled the paper over the exam table that crinkled under the pressure and sank down onto it until I was curled up tight on my side.

The world went hollow and distant. The PT said from miles away, "Better?"

"Worse," I said, the nothing in my stomach about to spew out everywhere. My heart beat hard enough to explode.

"We should try again," she said.

I wanted to yell, *No*. I wanted to fight back. Instead, I tried to cleave my mind from my body out of the clawing desperation that she somehow knew better than I did what I needed. I moved onto my back again, exposed. And then her hands and the whipping and the streaking sun slats. I curled up tighter on my side when it was over, the last ditch effort of protection from attacking bears and physical therapists.

"Sometimes this can last for a year or two." She shrugged a shoulder as if to say, *Sorry the jail cell is so small and there's only a nasty toilet in the corner, but at least there's three meals a day*.

Two years? My money was going to run out in about ten days. How was I going to interview for jobs? Maybe I could stretch the money I had left to fourteen days since I couldn't keep any food down anyway. My brain pounded through the options if this didn't go away soon, fear making it hard to swallow. Living with my mom was completely out of the question. I couldn't handle the stress and hardship of that relationship in addition to the stress and hardship of feeling this shitty every day. And then my mind dove into a blackness so complete I sucked in a breath to make sure I still could. The realization rose up like a slick, unscalable wall. I was in a relationship with someone I was certain wouldn't take care of me if I was this sick for that long. Our relationship was built on self-reliance, just like our life on that cold coastal beach.

My brother was in graduate school, living in a co-op. There was no one to lean on, and I wasn't a leaner anyway, I reminded myself as the physical therapist talked at me from some distant shoreline and I missed everything she said. I stayed curled up, tight and protected in that exposed space, and tried to find the energy I would need to deal with this on my own. How to find a job like this? Where to work? This was how it happened, I realized with clarity. A medical slide that led to sleeping in a car packed with all of your possessions.

CHAPTER TWO

My dad held court over a low fire on a muggy summer evening in 1983 in Missouri, one PBR in hand, many others zipping through his bloodstream. He was sitting in the grass next to the fire with my mom and his three best friends from growing up and their various assortment of girlfriends and wives. My dad, in his worn-out Levis and faded T-shirt, had everyone's attention.

I was supposed to be asleep, but it was hot inside Camp Sparkle, the falling down shack his buddies Adam, Coucher, and Davis had gone in together to buy on a sloping bank of a muddy river. Through the thin walls, the sound of my dad's laugh had me upright in bed, kicking free of the clawing sheet.

He was mercurial, some heaviness always pulling at him, but when he broke free, it was all sun and wide open skies, and I didn't like to miss it. I crept out of the bed I was sharing with my younger brother. It was nothing but a mattress on the floor, and I still had on the shorts and shirt I'd been wearing in the day. I moved through the dusty rooms and out into the thick night. The heavy air filled my lungs and grounded me. Made me know I was right where I was supposed to be. I found a tree just outside the circle of light the fire was putting off and settled in against the rough bark, where none of the adults would notice and tell me to go back to bed.

The firelight shaded my dad's face, eased the worry that lived there. He laughed again, easily, at something Davis said. He was in a storytelling mood. The kind that made me feel like life was one big adventure to be had. I settled in and waited. Beers always eased the path, being outside always helped, as did friends he didn't get to see often enough. It made him forget that we were constantly broke, that I left my shoes out in the living room like he hated, that I didn't want to eat anymore overgrown zucchini from the garden, even though that's what was for dinner, or that I'd kicked a hole in the drywall doing gymnastics in the house. He seemed happy when he told stories, and I craved the happy version of him.

Coucher, who, as far as I knew, only had the one name, said something I didn't fully catch about cops on a beach at night in Florida.

My dad laughed. A sound that filled me up. "Haven't seen you move that fast before or since," he said, taking a slug of beer.

"There were so many times we should've gotten arrested," Coucher said.

"Like the night we stole the donkey," Davis said.

My dad laughed again. I smiled, the warmth of the tree at my back, the smooth grass against my bare legs, as I imagined my high school dad and his friends stuffed into a beat up car with a donkey.

"And when you laid out your motorcycle in San Diego," my mom added.

"Hold up!" Coucher said. "I didn't hear that one. Let's have it! I need a beer first." He leaned over to the cooler. "Weaver?" he asked.

"Yep." My dad held up an open palm, and Coucher tossed him one.

"Anybody else?" Coucher asked. Once all the beers were distributed and my dad had guzzled what was left of the one and popped the top on the next, he squinted up like he did when recalling a story so he could tell it just right. "I was on my way home from work. Had this construction job. Ran a little errand on the way home." He smiled here, vaguely, just a flick at the corner of his lip, but a sure sign it was meant to be remembered. "And I was thinking about some bullshit the foreman had pulled that day and about how, soon enough, I wouldn't care, when some lady pulled out right in front of me. I'm cruising along, and then all of a sudden, I'm pile-driving into her rear windshield and then I'm flying over the top of her car. She hits the brakes and bounces me off the hood."

I saw it clearly. My dad's thin, muscled body rolling over the top of some old lady's car like Magnum PI. My mind put him in a leather motorcycle jacket, along with women on the sidewalk gasping as he hit the pavement, rolled to his feet, and gave them all a mustachioed smile.

"I wake up in the street with my leg all wrong and some dude leaning over me. I grabbed him by the collar like this." Dad reached over and got Adam by the neck of his T-shirt.

Adam shoved him off, and they toppled away from each other, laughing.

"Same leg you broke when you had that idea to ski in the dark because you're too cheap to buy a lift ticket?" Coucher asked.

"The other one," Dad said smiling. "Skiing in the daytime's for pansies, anyway," he added, further tattooing me with the understanding that adventure had a cost, and it was well worth it.

"So, I've got the guy by the collar." Firelight made it seem he was the only thing that existed in a sea of black. "I'm down on the ground, and I hear someone yelling, 'Call an ambulance,' and all I can think about is the big bag of weed in my jacket pocket."

"Shit!" Coucher yelled from the shadows.

"So this guy, I've got him by the shirt, and with my other hand, I reach into my jacket and stuff the bag of weed down his pants."

Everyone cracked up. "Why not down his shirt?" Davis asked through a laugh.

Dad flicked him a look as he cupped his hands and lit a cigarette. "It was all buttoned-up tight. He was some sort of business asshole. A tie, even."

"You changed a life!" Adam added.

"Did him some good," Dad agreed. "He walked off real quick."

On that night, and all the others when I listened to my dad dip into his past, I was being shaped by his words, the timing of his delivery, the images of him out there living outside the way we're expected to, of finding the back door when they won't let you in the front door because you aren't dressed right, don't know the right people, cuss too much.

"Here's the thing, Rach," he explained to me once as he, my brother, and I drove our purple boat of a car my great-grandmother had left to us fifteen miles an hour up the side of the highway all the way from Florida back to Tennessee. Something had broken, and a mechanic was out of the question when my dad could fix it for a fraction of the cost if we could just get it home to his tools. He was in that buzzy space between indulging the hot frustration over our current situation or laughing in the face of it, and I didn't want to do anything to shove him the wrong direction. He had one arm out his window, where he was waving cars past us since we were half in the highway. I sat in the front seat, and my brother was asleep on the couch of a back seat.

Dad looked over, cigarette in the corner of his mouth, one eye squinted up against the smoke. "If you expect your life to be easy like it is for those fuckers—" He waved a hand at the people whizzing by, presumably with enough money to buy nice cars that didn't break down on the way back from Florida, or with enough money to have them emergency fixed on a Sunday if they did. "Then you're going to be pissy all the time. Better to expect this kind of shit." He waved a hand to encompass the white, wispy smoke seeping out of the hood, the crumbling shoulder of the Georgia highway we bumped along as we made our slow way north. "Because it's gonna happen. It always does. You expect this, you'll learn how to handle it, and you'll be alright." His gaze moved back to the horizon as he inhaled on his cigarette, squinting up the one eye again. "If this thing catches fire," he added on the exhale, "be sure to shove your brother out on the side without the traffic."

In our house when I was growing up, life often felt like a minefield. But when he told stories, all that fell away. Life became something you could outsmart; having no money became something that sparked ingenuity and hilarity. No mood swings, no yelling, no quiet storms brewing. Only him at ease, the delight of a good story lived and told playing across his face, molding me into a shape that would prove unfit for marrying my high school boyfriend, buying a house, getting a proper job.

■ ■ ■

Three months into the all-the-time seasickness, a gooey fog settled permanently in my mind, making it hard to remember words, to string two ideas together, to remember what I was doing. Words continued to slide around on the page, as did cars in their lanes. Computers made me sick. So did rocking chairs and people who gesticulated while talking. I was dizzy in my dreams.

Because I needed to pass the courses I'd already paid for, because I'd just met the single mom and her four kids and it was unlikely I would find another rent-free situation, I began the practice of appearing as normal as possible. I dug in and pushed an impossibly big rock up an impossibly steep hill all day, every day, to do what I needed to do. I'd always been good in the face of immovable things.

I became two people: the one who looked fine at first glance, was a little quiet and blown-out, a little squinty and weird, but did what she was supposed to do. And then the other one who was crippled by fear and a world that wouldn't hold still, who didn't know who to talk to about it, or how, and so she quit trying.

The problem with all-the-time seasickness is that it had no outward signs. Unless you looked close enough to notice the glassy eyes, the way weight was falling off my already thin frame. Unless you paid attention to the fact that I was sleeping twelve hours each night, or to how hard it was for me to hold a conversation. I made simple meals for the family that fit the amount of energy it took to be upstairs and interacting: bad lentil soup, various versions of spaghetti, burritos. I had a full first draft of a novel written already, so I turned in old work, nodded and jotted down notes in workshop, and tucked away classmate's comments until some future point when I could actually read and incorporate them. I read the first page of each chapter of assigned texts to get the flavor of it and either kept my mouth closed or bullshitted my way through the discussion in class, aware that I was wasting massive amounts of money. But I wasn't living out of my car yet.

As it became more clear Karl wasn't going to move to Colorado for the summer, I entertained the idea of skipping the summer coursework and moving back to Alaska for the summer to work for the Forest Service again or to look for a job on a fishing boat. But as the weeks of landlocked seasickness went on, the idea of being able to function on a fishing boat or in the backcountry as a field tech stretched farther and farther away until I had to accept the reality of the jail cell with the nasty toilet as my only option until I could find the doctor who held the keys.

I endured weekly head whipping at the hands of the physical therapist. "It sometimes takes many treatments," she reassured me. I anxiously waited for the crystal to let go its death grip and fall back into place so I could have my life back. Each week, I continued to hand over my credit card because, despite the fact that I now had university insurance, because I'd seen the nurse practitioner before the insurance policy officially started, I had established the dizziness as a preexisting condition. Which meant no appointment treating me for dizziness would be covered for the first year of my insurance plan.

My credit card balance rolled over from three to four digits.

At the three-month mark, fear like ribbons wrapping and weaving my insides, I went back to the ENT. The first ENT I saw was now on vacation, so I saw his partner.

"It's not BPPV," I pleaded with him, trying to sit upright in the stupidly reclined chair. I needed to be assertive, make him see me, which wasn't possible with my belly exposed. "It's got to be something else because the Epley maneuver the PT has done four hundred times isn't working. What else can we try?" The edgy desperation in my own voice made me want to cry.

This ENT was an older man who smelled like recycled air. He sighed and stood up from the rolly chair. With impossibly soft hands, he stood in front of me and kneaded my neck up under my jawbone, held me still at the shoulder when he peered into my ear.

Afterward, he washed me off his hands in quick, efficient movements. His button-down shirt was pressed, as was his white doctor coat. I had grown used to wool and Carhartted men. Calloused hands and rough words.

The doctor popped the end of the ear instrument into the trash. "There's nothing wrong with your ears." He began to unscrew the top half of the ear instrument from the bottom half, fit them back into the small black case, his back still to me.

"If it's not my ears, what else could it be?"

He shrugged. Zippered the small black case closed.

"Have you considered therapy?"

I stared at him, my mouth hanging open, probably.

His face folded up into some sort of protective mask. "You know," he went on like I was six years old, "our bodies can react in severe ways to the daily stresses of life."

"I don't need therapy," I said. "Something is wrong. Biologically."

"Well," his voice clipped now, "there's nothing wrong with your ears."

This was not how medicine worked. This was not how my body worked. If anything went wrong, it righted itself, usually by itself, sometimes with a tidy prescription that took effect within twenty-four hours.

He reached out a hand for a shake. That soft, useless palm against mine. "Follow the hallway to your left to find your way out," he said as he swung open the door and walked off in the opposite direction.

I wanted to yell, *Wait!* I wanted to yell, *Help me!* I wanted to yell, *Please.* I closed my eyes and dropped my head to my forearm, curling up in the reclined chair. No one came in to ask me to leave or to see why I hadn't yet. They left me alone to ponder if this could possibly be some sort of jangly, repressed shit from my past, if I was going mad, if I was too weak to handle life's daily stresses.

■ ■ ■

"The ENT says it's not my ears," I explained to the momish nurse practitioner at her next available appointment. She had on a frumpy sweater and pressed slacks and seemed like someone I could trust.

She narrowed her brow. I watched her concentrate and thought, Yes, this is right. This is how it goes. We will discuss, she will ask questions that cannot be answered with yes or no. We will dig through the complicated layers until, together, we solve it. We will meet in the fertile ground of healing that exists between her medical knowledge and my precise explanation of what is happening inside my body.

"Okay," she breathed out, her hair a soft frizz all around her face. "Let's comb through the family history again, see if there is anything there." We went through all of it again, but I forgave her that, tried to see it as her way of stretching before the race started.

She sat there a moment. "How about any structural damage to your spine. Any recent falls? Something that maybe didn't seem like a big deal at the time?"

"I was a competitive gymnast growing up. I landed on my head a lot but nothing significant." I shrugged.

Her eyebrows flew up. She wrote something down.

"But that was such a long time ago," I added. "No car wrecks or significant falls in the past couple decades."

"Diet?" she asked.

"Whatever I could catch."

She squinted at me.

"Crab, halibut, salmon. I grew leafy greens in the summers."

"How much salmon?"

"A lot."

"Hmmm," she said. "We'll check mercury levels."

The walls of the exam room shimmered like curtains in a slight breeze. I tried to ignore them. I squinted to make them fuzzy. She ordered enough blood work that the tech had to go back for more vials. She ordered multiple X-rays to check for any structural irregularities in my spine.

My credit card bill blossomed.

■ ■ ■

In the week awaiting the results from all the tests, my phone rang as I pulled up to the house with the single mom, all the kids, and the dog that shed half itself every week.

"You haven't called in days." Karl's voice like a steamroller gaining speed.

"I'm so tired all the time." I took in all the cars smashed into the street, all the houses built on top of each other, the sound of someone's awful music, and missed the outdoor bathtub Karl and I had rigged up on the beach out of an old fish tote, several hoses, rainwater, and an on-demand hot water heater.

"You never think," he spat out, disgusted. "Have you even considered how that makes me feel?"

Once, I had backed out of the ferry car deck in a way that worked but was different than how he would've done it, which led to an all-out screaming match on the side of the road in Juneau. I often held the drill wrong or pulled the pull start wrong on the outboard. I didn't wash as many dishes as him, or feel sorry enough for what I'd done, or come home from the bar when he expected I should, or realize how I had actually hurt him.

The problem was, while I had moved to Alaska on my own, I couldn't afford to actually stay on my seasonal field tech's wage. I picked up winter work anytime I could find it, which wasn't often in a town of three thousand people, at least half of whom were out of work in the winter as well.

In order to keep the job I loved, I needed to share rent and food with someone else. I could've applied for a job with the city or at the grocery store and been able to continue living on my own in that small town I'd grown to love, but I wanted to fly around in float planes and hike around uninhabited islands all day, not bag groceries or sit at a desk.

When I spotted Karl competing in the logroll one Fourth of July, I thought, *Look at those abs!* He was living in an unheated, falling down shack at the end of the shipyard dock, and I was living in the attic of an old cannery. We got along well, he made me laugh, we loved the same things and, eventually, each other. When he landed a work trade, rent-free situation at an off the grid cabin out the road and asked me to join him, it seemed like the solution to all the problems.

Together, we could do what was not financially possible individually. We could live in the world's most perfect cabin on the ocean, without roommates. We could afford to rebuild a broken-down skiff by splitting the cost of the repairs, the trailer, and the shitty Evinrude. I did the simple work trade tasks, and he did the more complex ones, given his woodworking background. We fished my subsistence halibut license, soaked crab pots in front of our cabin, fished salmon at the nearby slough to fill the freezer and save on groceries. We cut standing dead, bucked it up, and hauled enough wood back to the cabin to provide heat through each winter. I tell myself now I could've gotten out, that building the life I so desperately wanted did not have to cost me his constant, slow chipping away of me, the degrading tone, the yelling on the docks and roadsides. But frogs in the pot coming to boil and all that. Once your life is built by balancing it against another, it's hard to find your way out of it, no matter how independent you think you are.

In my car that day in Colorado, on the phone, I listened to Karl elaborate about the injustice of me not putting him first, and after two years of trying a thousand different ways to extend the peaceful days between the fights, it suddenly seemed so simple. "Forget it," I interrupted him.

"What?" he said. I could hear the soft lap of the ocean in the background. I knew without asking that he was sitting on the small porch in one of the two comfortable chairs. Heard the smooth pull of rolling papers and the crinkle of the American Spirit bag, and I suddenly wanted a cigarette more than anything as I thought about how he would go on smoking a nightly cigarette on that narrow porch at the edge of the ocean and I never would again.

"I can't do this anymore." The dizziness simplified things into two distinct categories: what I could do and what I couldn't do.

"You don't mean that," he said.

I wasn't sure who was demanding it, me or the dizziness, but I knew it was not possible to be beat down any more than I already was. Suddenly, the life we'd build wasn't worth hanging onto at this price. "I'm done."

There was more to it—some ugly words. I hung up the phone, sat in the driver's seat with the chaos of the world closing in around me, dazed by the fact that I'd just sliced myself free of Alaska and the person I was closest to in the world.

■ ■ ■

Two days later, in the nurse practitioner's office, she said, "Here, take a look at the X-ray." On the backlit screen, she hung up the

butterfly image of my torso, and I wanted to yank it down immediately. I had always been so strong, so independent, and here
was proof that I was nothing but whispery, small bones, the rest
of my body fading into nothing in the background. She pointed.
"No irregularities in your backbone," she explained. "All your blood
work came back normal. You are actually one of the healthiest
thirty-one-year-olds I've seen in a while." She shook her head. The
defeated angle of it set my teeth on edge.

"But there's clearly something wrong." I was pleading, trying
to shove myself in the way of the door that seemed to be swinging shut between us. I needed a partner. One who believed I was
sick. One who knew more than I did about medical solutions.
Someone who would not give up on me.

She didn't say anything, just sighed.

"What's the next step?" I pushed.

She shrugged. "CoQ10 is a supplement that helps with a wide
variety of things. You could try that. It's expensive though."

She sat on the rolly thing but suddenly began stretching farther and farther away from me in my vision in some sort of Alice
in Wonderland phenomenon. This hadn't happened before. The
dizziness was alive and growing new appendages, gaining new
skills. I shut my eyes tight.

She touched my knee and said gently, "I really think it's just
stress." The door between us slammed shut.

Because I didn't want to cry in front of her, I gathered up my
things. I walked down the slanted funhouse hallway and out into
the blaring sunshine. Because my car was the only quiet place in
my life, I sat in it for a long time. I watched a younger, lighter

version of myself walk by, hand in hand with her boyfriend as they crossed campus. I watched the way she tossed her head back in laughter, the easy set to her shoulders.

I was afraid to cry. Afraid that if I started, I would never stop.

I'd survived so much: the constant dull roar of poverty with no safety net, a shipwreck, Cuban pirates, a dynamite incident in Croatia, charging bears, bush planes diving toward the earth on stormy days. It wasn't stress. It was a biological malfunction. I wasn't imagining it. It wasn't a matter of deep breathing and clear thinking to gain control over it. No amount of talking about my feelings to a therapist was going to stop the floors from sloshing. I needed pharmaceuticals. I needed answers. I needed to find someone who believed me.

I had stepped through the front door of the medical system without questioning that I would be guided toward a solution by smart, competent, caring people as long as I was a smart, competent, compliant patient. I had not imagined the shrugs, the platitudes, the desperate act of trying to convince them that there was actually something wrong with me. Where were the doctors who didn't give up, who dug in and tried and tried and tried until whatever was wrong was no longer wrong? I had always assumed doctors were like pond ice in the dead of winter. Solid, able to hold the weight of a skater or a truck.

More clarity descended: To be this dizzy for much longer would lead to total collapse. If I couldn't work, couldn't support myself, then what? My car was paid off. The seats reclined nicely. I could live in it for a short period of time at least. I closed my eyes, tried to swallow the fear that clawed in my throat. I would find the doctor who was willing to make the long walk to the middle where we could compare notes. I would get better at reporting the intricacies of the sick world, he or she or they would bring their vast knowledge from the medical world, we would pull up chairs, put our heads together, and find a solution. I just had to keep going until I found that doctor. Or possibly, more simply, I just had to randomly land on the doctor who had seen what I had before, without the help of a famous dad doctor with doctor buddies and without the cash to fly all around to the top institutions in the world. Good fucking luck, younger me.

CHAPTER THREE

Because everything jumped and swam in my vision, I googled ophthalmologists who specialized in weird issues. If it wasn't my ears, this seemed a likely solution. Maybe I just needed new glasses? Fuck, that would be fantastic.

The computer screen sent the dizziness into overdrive. In my tiny basement room, the wall, the desk, the lamp lurched and swung. I lasted about three minutes. I held onto the desk, tried to absorb as much as I could on the screen before I had to close my eyes. I slid down to the floor, willing my mind to meld with the floor's solidity.

I lay on the carpet, breathing hard, as if I'd just survived something. The room rocked and swayed beneath me for the next half hour. As it began to ease, I slowly raised myself back into the chair, closed one eye to be able to line up the mouse with the name at the top of the Google search, called, and made an appointment.

In the next two three-minute spurts, I looked into buying other insurance, but no matter where I went, the preexisting condition would follow and I would continue to pay out of pocket.

■ ■ ■

Ten days later, at the ophthalmologist's first available appointment, I settled into the vaguely reclined, padded chair in the middle of the exam room and answered all the questions about symptoms, onset, and past medical history. While she typed everything into the computer, her back to me, I checked out the pictures on the wall and felt heartened by the goats. In the picture closest to me, the doctor was bent, one knee on the ground, her arms looped around an indifferent goat's neck. Perhaps she was someone who cared indiscriminately.

Eventually, she turned from the computer and stood in front of me. She flipped off the overhead light, which shaved one corner off the dizziness. She asked me to follow her finger while covering one of my eyes with a wide black spoon, which was basically impossible.

"Your eyes will not track or converge," she said, looking at me directly now, her long, loose, gray hair framing her face. "I'll bet you feel terrible."

"Pretty terrible," I said, so grateful I wanted to cry.

"We address an issue like this with vision therapy." Her face expressed confidence, caring, and authority. "You'll need to come in twice a week for at least three months. And you'll have daily exercises. Don't expect much improvement before that three-month mark. It's important to stick with the therapy in order to get the cumulative effect."

She turned toward the door, clearly oblivious to the fact that she'd just condemned me to three more months of struggling through every minute of every hour of every day, and to multiple appointments per week that were going to be well outside my financial reach. Shame filled me. I'd been putting off the job search until I could walk down hallways without dragging a finger against a wall to know where it was. For the vast majority of my life, I'd held no less than two jobs at all times. I wanted to explain to her that I needed this taken care of today, not in three months, that there was no time or safe place to curl up and do eye exercises until I started to feel better.

The doctor spun for the door. "You can make your first set of appointments with Cindy up front."

I forced a smile. "Thank you."

■ ■ ■

Vision therapy took place in a room with kid sized chairs. Amy, the vision therapist, sat down across from me at a kid sized table. While it was weird, it was also nice to be closer to the ground. *Maybe they know what they're doing. Maybe there are a lot of dizzy people who come here to be cured on kindergarten furniture.* Amy, the cheerful woman who presided over the room full of bouncy balls and string, handed me a yardstick with three pushpins along its length. "Hold this out in front of your face like this." She was one of those friendly shaped women. Soft everywhere, with deep wrinkles at the edges of her mouth and eyes.

I imitated her and settled the yardstick into the notch of my shoulder, where the butt of the shotgun used to rest.

"Great," she said in the tone of a patient teacher. "Now, settle your eyes as best you can on the farthest away pushpin. When I say now, move them quickly to the middle pin, and when I say now again, move them to the closest pin. Ready?" She picked up the stopwatch that was hanging around her neck and pushed her glasses up her nose.

"Sure," I said, settling my eyes on the farthest pin, wondering what I was doing. I thought, *This is ridiculous, I should leave now*. I flicked my eyes over to the door. It wasn't far, but the floor between me and the door rolled like an ocean swell. It seemed easier to stay where I was than to try to walk up and over it. I refocused on the farthest away pushpin and told myself that they'd treated this before. That moving my eyes from one pushpin to another was for sure going to right the world.

"Now," Amy said. I moved my eyes to the middle pushpin, and the room flipped over. I dropped the yardstick and held onto the small table. Desperation blacked out everything else. If I couldn't move my eyes a one-foot distance, how was I going to feed myself?

Amy was at my side, an arm over my shoulders. "Okay, okay," she was saying from a watery distance away. "Sometimes it's hard at first, but it gets easier. Let's take a break. Want some water?"

I made some noise she took to be a yes, and she left me for a minute. I curled up on the floor and covered my head with my arms. It wasn't news to me that something that was supposed to make you better had to make you worse first. I just didn't know how much worse I could handle it getting.

After a miniature waxy cup of water and two more tries, Amy called it a day. "Let's get you to the calm down room."

She led me to a dark closet, empty but for a chair and one pinprick of light against one wall. Amy smiled so big that her cheeks lifted her glasses up. "When I close this door, it's going to be very dark. Stare at the light to help bring back the lost equilibrium in your vision." She backed out on tiptoe and closed the door as if I were a sleeping child she didn't want to wake. Once I was enveloped in darkness, my shoulders relaxed. While the perfectly still pinprick jigged and jagged in my vision, the soundless, pitch-black room stilled something deep inside me. While the family I lived with was turning out to be lovely, four kids are always in motion, always hungry, always loud, making me physically ache for a canopy of two-hundred-year-old trees locked in an embrace, a forest floor blanketed with moss, a constant cloud bank comfortably close overhead. I put myself back on the porch in the white chair, wrapped in a sleeping bag as I'd spent so many evenings, listening to the lap of ocean, the hiss of rain, the sound of both almost reaching me in the small, dark closet.

■ ■ ■

On a humid night in April of 1992 I was counting calories, only allowing myself to buy a Blow Pop at a high school soccer game, when the mom on the other side of the folding table that served as a concession stand grabbed my wrist. Her thick red fingernails locked together, holding me still but not squeezing. She caught my eyes in that one moment I had left, holding off what she knew was coming next for as long as she could.

And then her face crumpled. "Your father," she said. We didn't know each other except in the way you do in small southern towns. Our lives linked in ways as thin and strong as a spider's web. "Mrs. Jordan is looking for you."

As if on cue, my friend Ben's mom appeared, her arm loosely around me, directing me toward the parking lot behind the bleachers. Something had happened out at the ballfields, and it had to do with my dad. As the paramedics worked to thrust life back into his chest, someone had been dispatched to collect my brother and me from the high school, and Mrs. Jordan had taken it from there. At that point, I didn't know my dad lay in the dust of the chalky line between home and first, but I'd heard the ambulance go screaming by. We all had.

My brother had been gathered up by Mr. Jordan. Matt appeared at my side, twiggy and big, headed in the way of freshman boys. He wasn't saying anything either.

"We'll drive you to the hospital," Mrs. Jordan said, her tiny waist accented by a wide elastic belt. Mr. and Mrs. Jordan were watching my brother and me closely. My skin prickled. They rushed us into the dimly lit parking lot, them in a hurry, me trying to hold us back from whatever we were rushing toward.

"I'll drive," I said. Even then, I knew to snatch and hold tight to any semblance of normality as a way to convince yourself and others that you are not falling apart.

Mrs. Jordan met my eyes.

"What happened?" I managed to ask in half a whisper.

Before she flicked her gaze away, they filled with a sorrow thick as the night we had plunged into. "We have to go. Your mom is at the ER." She scanned the parking lot for my car and then directed all four of us toward it. "I'll ride with you."

We rushed into the ER waiting room packed full of my dad's office softball teammates dressed in their matching T-shirts. Several looked down immediately, others began to fidget. A man was crying silently. No one said anything as one of the nurses disappeared into the back to get my mom. My brother and I and the Jordans stood in the middle of the room for an awkward few seconds before my mom rushed out from behind a swinging door. She took us outside to tell us, as if that would be easier. We stood in the parking lot, cushioned by the humid night under a thousand stars. "He's gone," she said, and so was I.

■ ■ ■

Three months into the all-the-time seasickness, I found a job posting for a second shift at an aerospace company that involved working with liquid nitrogen, the stuff doctors use to burn moles off. Just out of college, I'd worked in a chemistry lab, where I'd mastered the skill of avoiding burns while filling the Carlo Rossi-looking jugs I was meant to fill with liquid nitrogen. I'd also mastered creating a smoky dance floor in one of the back rooms and freezing flowers I'd picked outside to smash into a million pieces on the countertop.

While I had unlimited skills with liquid nitrogen, I had no skills in aerospace engineering. All I knew was that I needed money, and this job paid well, and a second shift meant I could go to school in the day and still work full time. I held as still as possible in the chair, kept my hands clasped in my lap, and hoped the two men interviewing me would not notice that I swayed in a wind that wasn't there. Or how desperate I was for a part-time job that was likely to turn into a full-time job that came with the promise of health insurance after a six-month trial period.

The older man who was leading the interview leaned over my résumé on the slick-topped table. His white hair was gelled into place, and he had a body that looked to be perpetually hunched in front of a screen. He sent a piercing look across the table. "Would you say you are comfortable working in a male dominated work environment?" He narrowed his eyes in challenge, but he was still hunched, clearly unaware of his submissive posture.

The younger man who had told me, when he greeted me at the front door, that he'd spent part of his childhood in Anchorage said, "She worked in the backcountry of Alaska. She'll be fine here."

I thought of the work I'd done collaring bears with the unpredictable Vietnam vet with electric white hair, who had once shot a bear while it was on top of him. Of the time a drunk fisherman, who thought it might be just the thing to win me over, ran across the bar, threw me over his shoulder, tossed me in a van, and drove me twenty miles out the road where there was nothing but wind and waves, dense forest, and other drunk men.

I arranged my face to suggest that I understood the concern of working with a bunch of carefully scrubbed and gelled aerospace engineers. "I can handle myself in male dominated situations."

"Can you explain the nature of the work you did? What was it? With the Forest Service?" the older man asked me. I talked for a few minutes about boats and rifles and helicopters. Of long days climbing steep mountains with a heavy pack, camping, and bears. I blinked rapidly at the tears forming as the realization descended that in my current state, it would be impossible for me to do a single thing I was describing. As I painted that colorful life with words in a sterile boardroom, it stretched out of reach, and I understood for the first time that it might stay that way. I blinked a couple more times, pretended something was in my eye.

The men hired me. A week later, as I was filling out paperwork in the office of an impressively thin, single mom HR representative, I closed one eye to get the room to hold still as much as possible and said, "So, the insurance?"

"Yeah?" she said. She sat in her chair across the wide desk with one foot tucked up underneath her, blonde hair curling in big ringlets around her face and shoulders.

"They don't have any preexisting clauses, do they?"

"Let's see," she said in the cheery way of someone who has never had to wonder such a thing. She scrolled and typed and then said, "Looks like they will cover preexisting conditions after you've paid monthly premiums for six months." She looked up. "But your job is part time. Only full-time employees are offered health insurance." Which I knew of course, but it flayed me to hear this latest failure stated outright. Competent, smart, in-demand people are offered full-time jobs.

"Right." I held my breath to keep from crying. "Thanks," I managed to get out.

As I walked the hallway, I kept my eyes on the top corner of the ceiling to keep the repeating pattern on the carpet out of my peripheral view. I told myself I'd do whatever it took to make the men move me to full time as soon as possible. The pay was unbelievable at part time. The pay at full time, with the promise of insurance in six months, would solve everything.

The quickest way to full-time work was to appear as normal as possible. During my shifts, I made up interruptions to get off the computer at the three-minute mark, memorized directions for test chambers so I only had to read them once, wore noise cancelling headphones to block out the overwhelming sound of it all.

I practiced compartmentalizing the all day seasickness, the nausea, the exhaustion. I imagined them like thick, wooden blocks, the kind kids play with, stacked up off to the side in my brain. I stayed focused on the possibility of insurance with no restrictions and the plan to put myself in front of as many clinicians as I could find until someone recognized what was wrong or was willing to help for long enough to help me figure it out.

I paced to stay awake until my shift ended at midnight, ignored the way my body begged for more sleep, ignored how hard it was to appear normal, fiercely concentrated all day long to see through the brain fog. Each month, I belted my loosening pair of jeans tighter.

■ ■ ■

With my first paycheck in the bank, I decided to splurge on a frothy coffee. I stepped into a busy coffee shop.

"No way," a voice I recognized from some other life said. "Thought you were in Alaska." Mike stood up and gave me a hug.

I wasn't dead. I couldn't help but notice the ropy arms and wide chest. The spark in his eyes as he said, "You remember Dan," pointing at the man he was having coffee with. "He's married." I laughed. A sound so startling, I covered my mouth. Ten years previous, most of the women I hung out with had either dated or hoped to date Dan.

"Are you back?" Mike asked.

"Grad school," I said. And then, because I didn't want to explain any other part of the situation, I followed up with, "Still with the fire department?"

"Seven years now." He slid his hands into his pockets. "Want to catch up sometime? Go out for a beer?" he grinned.

"I'd love to," I said.

As if I could drink a beer.

■ ■ ■

The next day, Mike left a message on my phone: "Here's my phone number. I hope you'll . . . use it."

I laughed and called him back. We met for a burger and beer, although I drank water. In his steady presence, I felt calm for the first time since I'd left my cushy white chair on my porch, the soft sound of water on a closed up Alaskan night. I felt for the first time lifted out of the dizziness back into life where you chat about what you've been up to, laugh together in a crowded pub, stroll leisurely through all the common ground between yourself and another person.

■ ■ ■

At the end of three months of vision therapy, I wasn't any better. I sat in the ophthalmologist's chair and, this time, noticed how neither she nor the goat actually looked comfortable in the picture. Something about the awkward angle of her elbow, the dip of the goat shoulders away from her embrace. "Sorry," she said from her roll chair, and I knew she meant it. "It's not your eyes."

"What do you think it is then?"

"I couldn't say." She looked tired.

"If you had to guess." I was way more tired than she was.

"It's not your eyes," she said a little more forcefully. "Probably just anxiety. An antidepressant might help."

I closed my eyes. "If it's not my ocular system, what other biological," I paused here for emphasis, "issue could be causing things to jump around in my vision?"

"It's not your eyes," she said again in a tone you use with a kid you are done with who wants to continue arguing.

I wanted to scream, *But you are the one who went to medical school!* Wasn't she supposed to be interested in solving complex biological problems? Didn't she study the whole body before specializing in eyes?

Instead, I gathered my bag and left, wondering if perhaps it wasn't an interest in solving complex biological problems but more an interest in owning enough land to raise goats.

That afternoon, I gathered up my courage, crept up sideways on the computer like it was full of venom, and searched for neurologists. If it wasn't my ears or my eyes, perhaps it was my brain. I read what I could and then squeezed my eyes tight as I lay on the floor that moved like my sixteen-foot skiff when the Evinrude crapped out in big water. Minus the amazing landscape.

I needed someone who would listen. I needed someone who would spend the time thinking instead of fussing with the mouse. Someone who would take some time to hear and discuss rather than someone who scheduled five appointments per hour.

When I gathered up my courage to look at the screen again, one of the links read "Holistic Neurology." When I clicked on it, I caught "One-Hour Appointments." I called and asked for the first available appointment.

■ ■ ■

On the first anniversary of Dad's death, there were curtains of lightning. Bright flashes every few seconds, the smell of things burning, the weight of rain in my clothes as I ran for cover. The power of the storm a force against my body, as if he were reaching through the void, trying to say something. There were a lot of things that needed saying: Stop drinking so much. Start caring about something. Don't fuck up your whole life at the age of eighteen.

On the second anniversary of his death, there was wind strong enough to spiderweb windshields as I sprinted across campus, late for the class I was failing. My dad's coworkers had passed around a baseball hat and collected enough cash to pay for several classes at the college down the road.

On the third anniversary, I was, quite randomly, living aboard a 130-foot wooden boat. My mom had come home with a book from the library that had long lists of adventurous ways to earn college credit. She flipped it open and pointed at a sail training program. I pointed at the tuition, which was ten times the cost of the college I was currently attending.

"Look at what it costs!" I said. Never mind that I'd never been out in the ocean on a boat before. Or that I got seasick on swings.

"You'll get a scholarship." She snapped the book closed. "We're broke, and you're a mess."

I got a scholarship. Along with nineteen other students, I spent two months in Woods Hole, Massachusetts, learning celestial navigation, studying oceanography and the history of seafaring, and then flew to Miami to board the boat with ten faculty. For weeks, hundreds of miles out of sight of any land, we'd been in constant thirty-foot waves and steady winds.

Most people puked the first few days out and then got over it. One guy was seasick the whole time. Two of us didn't get seasick at all.

On the morning of the third anniversary of my dad's death, we woke up to flat, eerie calm in the South Sargasso Sea. No wind, not a ripple in the water. We were forced to float, to wait, to hold. After so much motion, it was unnerving.

We wandered about, applied more sunscreen, baked in the relentless sun, and watched the captain shake his head. Doldrums weren't common in this area.

Betsy was another student onboard. I was nineteen to her twenty-one, she'd lost her dad at the age of sixteen. Her father was a dentist who made jewelry in his spare time.

He'd crafted her a necklace by hand shortly before he died, a small bronze sun with rays casting out of the center haphazardly. She wore it around her neck at all times. She was the first person

I'd met whose father had also dropped dead of a sudden and massive heart attack, leaving her in that vast, slippery space I recognized, where there was nothing to hold onto.

We spent that whole listless afternoon tucked up against stored away sails, talking about things other than who to hook up with, how much beer we liked to drink, what college we went to and how much fun it was.

The wind began to pick up again in the evening of the doldrum day, slow and steady until we were back in thirty-foot waves, the boat and all of us in constant motion. We had all learned celestial navigation and used a small, wooden chart table to plot out our course based on sextant measurements taken at sunrise, noon, and sunset every day.

I woke up for my 3:00 a.m. shift, sat up, and reached for the chart table to steady myself as I got to my feet. Betsy's necklace was there on top of the chart. I grabbed it, afraid it would be flung into oblivion with the next roll of the wave.

I knew Betsy was now asleep in a bunk near the bow of the boat. The sailing of the boat was divided up into three shifts. She was on C shift and would take over for me and the rest of my group at 7:00 a.m. It must've come off when she figured our position at some point on her last shift. I zippered the necklace in the pocket of my shorts and headed up the four stairs to the aft deck.

As I steered by compass at the large, wooden spoked wheel through the blue night under a thousand stars, I felt sick with the possibility that she might have lost the last thing her father had given her. I had nothing tangible like that. My father's buddy owned a rickety, small boat they liked to sail around a small, hot lake on the weekends. He had offered up a smile as I walked out the door less than an hour before he died. "Want to go sailing tomorrow, bub?"

At 7:00 a.m., Betsy came up the stairs bleary eyed, her brown hair a disaster of sleep. "Bets!" I called. "Your necklace." I held it out in my palm.

Her hand went to her neck immediately, where her necklace was securely fastened. The bright morning sun lit one half of her wide face and threw a shadow over the rest. Her dark eyes caught mine. She picked up the small bronze medallion I still held out in my hand. It was a round sun, thick rays branching off, a small circle at the top to loop a thin strap of leather or twine through. She looked up. "It's like mine, but it's not mine." She held up the one around her neck so I could compare the two. The one I'd found was a bit smaller, a bit more delicate, the branching of the sun rays was different.

"I've never seen that one before," she said, her voice catching as she placed it back in my hand.

I felt cold despite the warm breeze. The dark sea rose and fell, the surface of the water glinted as I closed my fingers over the small sun.

We asked every single person on board. No one had brought it, no one had seen it before, and no one had noticed it on the chart table throughout the hourly check of our current location in the shift before mine.

I found a thin length of rope on the boat and hung the sun around my neck.

On a morning toward the end of my time on the sailboat, as I was brushing my teeth at the tiny bathroom sink, feet and elbows wedged to keep me upright in the particularly large rollers, I realized I didn't have to be, first and foremost, the sad girl whose dad just died. I froze in front of the mirror smeared with salty water residue, the toothpaste burning my tongue and dripping from my bottom lip, my whole body tingling with the realization that instead of holding this sadness up in between myself and the world, I could use it to propel myself toward my own adventures. I rinsed my mouth and face with salt water from the tap and finished up my small, personal, miraculous discovery in a hot, metallic bathroom fifty miles out at sea. I knew three things to be true:

First, nothing could be counted on. If you could laugh and joke with the dad you so desperately needed to stay in your life on your way to a high school soccer game and, one hour later, he was dead, how could you ever see life as anything more than untrustworthy? If I settled back in, let down my guard, and started to trust, I'd get blindsided again. I needed to be ready for the next left hook. I needed to stay on my toes, keep uncertainty close so that I was always expecting it.

Second, it was better to love fewer people so there was less to lose.

Third, I wouldn't make it past forty-five years old either. This one is harder to explain. I was a logical person, but this seemed inevitable. It had to do with the knowledge I was more like my dad than not. There was no autopsy. There was an offhand comment by my mom that it was likely some genetic problem with his heart. It wasn't that I knew we had the same heart condition; it was that I knew we had the same heart.

And so, a couple days after I got back home from the semester on the boat, I packed up my car and folded the eighty dollars I had to my name into the ashtray. I pulled out of the small town in Tennessee I'd grown up in and pointed myself toward Colorado, the sun still tied around my neck.

I wanted wide open spaces, something new, something unexpected, wild lands to stress-test me, to keep me ready and well practiced for the next calamity life would deal me.

I had no credit card, no cell phone. I had a tent, a map, and a fishing pole. I drove into the forever setting sun and eventually made it to Colorado hungry and running on adrenaline, imagining how my dad would tell it around a campfire.

■ ■ ■

I dropped my month-long summer class. There was no point. I drove the one hour to the holistic neurologist. I kept one eye closed, and yet, cars shimmered in their lanes and occasionally leapt wildly toward me. I tightened the muscles in my back, my grip on the wheel. Willed myself not to swerve away because it was all in my head. Cars do not jump sideways off the pavement. They were in their lane, and I was in mine. I wondered if I was losing my mind. I wondered if this was all my own doing. If I had used my life to stress test myself to the point of snapping in two. I should've settled into the perceived safety of driving to work, sitting in a cubicle, decorating for Christmas. The kind of life that doesn't tax your nervous system with huge dumps of adrenaline when the Cessna is dropping toward earth or in that moment when the bear shifts from curious to mad. Perhaps if I could've weathered my dad's death better, I could've handled my relationship with my mom better instead of being cut raw by both. If I'd chosen different men to date, hadn't gone to the logroll competition, hadn't chased this stupid dream of writing books. Maybe I did need an antidepressant. Or better yet, some sort of make-better-life-decisions-you-freaking-idiot pill.

As traffic slowed to a standstill, I knew with certainty that the neurologist would tell me I had a brain tumor. What then? Let it grow while I talked my way into full-time work and waited out the six months of premiums until my health insurance would cover a surgery to remove it? What if I didn't live that long? Is this the inky underbelly of how it all works? If you have money, you can take care of the brain tumor, if you don't, oh well? A hushed up cleaning out of the people who can't or don't plug into white collared America?

I feel the need to take a minute to say I am not a delinquent. I have always had a job or two or three, never carried a balance on my credit card until the world started spinning. I paid off my undergraduate student loans in under a decade by eating a lot of toast. In the years of working for the Forest Service, which did not offer health insurance to seasonal employees, I paid for catastrophic health insurance and considered myself responsible in maintaining the added expense. I drove cars I had paid outright for (sometimes the outright was $500, but still, no car loans), I traveled in Europe not by spending money but by getting a job on a sailboat as crew. I had never borrowed money from anyone, ever. I had always figured it out. Until my situation became impossible to figure out.

The neurologist had a cozy waiting room. The chairs were actual cloth, and the lamps gave off cones of warm light. As I collapsed into the soft chair and let the easy light soothe the terrible car ride out of my system, I had the thought that this room alone was worth the $100 per fifteen minutes I was about to spend. The holistic neurologist herself came out to usher me into the exam room. She had blonde, kinky hair and a serious manner. She was tiny, dressed in a sweater despite the summer heat. She looked too small to hold the burden of my situation. Too cold to be able to focus well. She asked me to undress and put on the thin cotton contraption of hospitals. "Open in the back, please," she called out as she left the exam room.

Once I was ready, the neurologist performed a slow, laborious examination, in which I had to walk and balance and follow her finger with my eyes. Not a single thing that required a thin cotton gown that opened in the back. The room was exceptionally cold. I began to shiver. Her hands were ice. She ran the cold metal end of the reflex hammer along the bottom of my foot. It tickled, and I jumped. "Hmmm . . ." she said. She did it again. This time, I was expecting it and did not jump. I was excessively ticklish as a kid but had learned to mind-over-matter it as I grew up. Unless I was caught by surprise.

"That's strange," she said.

As a biology major in college, I had been in class with many people who had gone on to medical school. Most of them fit the profile: nervous knees, plenty of sharpened number twos. But for all the curve setting, there was often an alarming lack of common sense.

The neurologist ran the blunt end of the hammer along the bottom of my foot a third time. Nothing.

I looked up, expecting some conversation. But I was a body, not a person. I was a complex conglomeration of nerves and brain and muscles that were not acting right. "What is it?" I asked, finally.

She looked up, startled to see me.

"Your foot. It's unusual."

I looked at my bare foot, slightly blue now, given the cold room. "The way it jumped?" I asked. She was frowning, looking down at my foot.

"An MRI might not be a bad idea," she said.

"To look for what?"

"A brain tumor."

My heart constricted. It would make sense. The thick fog my brain had turned into. The hurricane of the world around me. But what did a ticklish foot have to do with it?

"My insurance won't cover an MRI, and I don't have the money for it unless you feel certain it is necessary, in which case, I'll come up with the money somehow. What is your suspicion of a brain tumor based on?"

She began to close up. Her face first, then her body. She took a step away. She used a bunch of big words and pointed to my foot. "It's unusual."

"It tickled," I countered. I didn't want a brain tumor. I wanted a discussion. I wanted more proof that I should spend thousands of dollars on an MRI. I needed her to slow down, to explain it in a way that my broken brain could fully understand.

Something flickered across her face that I couldn't read. Frustration, it seemed. "I'm not saying it was anything definitive," she snapped. "I'm just saying it would be in your best interest to rule out the big stuff. Throw your smock in the dirty clothes bin there." She pointed and was gone. The distance between the land of the sick and the land of the well too great to overcome. The clock struck one hour.

I dropped my head. It was too much to explain. Every conversation searching for the right words sapped energy I didn't have. Even my bones felt tired. I wasn't trying to be combative or to make her do all the work. I was pinned down in sick land, trying to keep the desperation of dizziness and lack of money from strangling me in front of her.

CHAPTER FOUR

That afternoon, at home in my basement room with a herd of elephant teenagers overhead, I looked up how much an MRI cost out of pocket. An impossible number in the thousands. I laid my head in the crook of my arm and granted permission to feel sorry for myself. A slippery slope that typically ended in a blackout where life didn't seem worth it. Dangerous unless I set a timer. I set it for five minutes, and 100 percent wallowed until I had to go to work. It physically hurt to stay up until midnight. I struggled through those late night hours at the lab when time slowed down and I didn't have much to do, my dizzy mind and exhausted body begging for sleep.

The company I worked for was building pieces and parts that would go up on satellites and the next Mars rover. My job was to run vacuum chambers that simulated space-like conditions of temperature and pressure. The engineers would design the parts, the machinists would build them, the mechanism would go into the vacuum chambers where I and the other test technicians would simulate the temperature changes the mechanism was likely to see in space twenty-four hours a day for weeks on end.

At certain points in the testing cycle, a build technician would come in to test the piece to make sure it could do what it was supposed to do when under the extremes of space-like temps and pressures. What this meant was that every thirty minutes, I adjusted the temperature and made sure the chamber was holding a vacuum correctly. By the time the piece got to the test center, it was often worth a lot of money. Every once in a while, I would hear how much it was worth and then wish I didn't know. If it saw one degree too high or too low in the temperature spectrum, it was often ruined.

My job was mostly to make sure everything was fine and to be around to do something if it was not. As long as the chambers were working as they were supposed to, I had twenty-eight minutes in between chamber checks to stare at the cubical wall while wearing my noise cancelling headphones. Mostly to cancel out all the clicking and whooshing and high-pitched squealing that made my head pound. And secondarily, to cancel out anyone's inclination to come talk to me. I had nothing good to say and no extra energy to hold polite conversations.

That particular night, after the holistic neurologist appointment, I spent each of my twenty-eight-minute breaks trying to figure out if I needed an MRI. I jumped because I was ticklish, surely. But what did I know of the dark recesses of neurology? Not much. But how much did she know? I thought of all the people who had likely sat in her exam room who never thought twice about scheduling the recommended MRI that would require nothing more than a $100 copay and an uncomfortable hour in the tube.

I wrote down the temps on the half hour, 10:30 p.m., and sunk back into my cubicle. I wanted wind and water and the adventure of a flight the next day to a densely forested island man had yet to mess up, where I'd spend all day trying to flush out a male goshawk with a recorded territorial call. I wanted nothing more than to have the physical ability to track him all day, up and over fallen hemlocks, through squishy muskegs, up steep hillsides, back to his nest that I would mark on the map and keep the timber crews from cutting down. I slowly removed myself from the loud lab in the middle of the country in the middle of the night until I could almost, almost feel the misty rain on my face, the heavy air filling my lungs.

I opened my eyes to a spinning, dusty, concrete lab clicking and clacking with manmade bullshit to help Home Depot track packages shipped from China to Oklahoma and suddenly felt like I was drowning.

I stood up, frantic to pull myself out. I paced. I looked at the pictures of wives and girlfriends in other people's empty cubicles, started imagining the details of their lives based on the Snickers wrappers in their trash and the things tacked up on their cubicle walls. Once I'd given one guy a sordid past of honky tonks and arm wrestling championships, and another a prep school accidental pregnancy with the mysterious girl from algebra, my shoulder blades began to ease back to their rightful places. I'd always enjoyed making things up but suddenly saw it clearly for the refuge it was. The only way out of the jail cell. My mind slid into the world of my novel I'd abandoned working on with the onset of the dizziness seven months prior.

As I walked the long concrete corridor of cubicles, the high-ceilinged warehouse dim with the night, I let my mind step aboard the fishing boat of the brothers I had given beards and an easy way with each other. I sank in deeper and felt the ease in the body of my main character, Ellie, who could haul in fish as the brothers' crew, shoot off witty comebacks, and keep her balance as nasty storms raged all around.

I swung by the copier, stole some blank paper, walked back over to my desk, closed my eyes, and started on page one of the story that was already written. Dealing with edits in a Word doc was not possible; nor was reading. I'd listened and absorbed the advice my classmates and professors had given me when my pages were discussed but had felt hog tied as far as how to implement those changes with the dizziness in the way. If I couldn't go back in, I'd start over.

I put myself back in the land of glaciers and dark, huge trees as far as the eye could see, of night skies full of arcing northern lights, of water and gulls and bears and rain. I started at the beginning, where I'd started a year and a half prior, wrapped up in my sleeping bag on the porch of my cabin.

At my desk, I wrote with my eyes closed until the pen hit the slick surface of the desk at the edge of the page. Each time, I took a quick glance to set my pen in the right place for the next line and kept going. Time fell away, and the dark nothingness let go its awful pull. I got a full breath of air for the first time in months.

■ ■ ■

Acupuncture, I'd heard, works wonders.

I found an established practitioner and made an appointment. She wore flowy clothes and took notes by hand, no computer in sight. She looked into my eyes as I told her the dizzy story, and she didn't interrupt. Her brow furrowed in what looked to be true concern. The room was dimly lit, there was the soft sound of a waterfall in the background, and the shade slats were pulled mercifully closed.

She asked about my life and my symptoms, nodding her head, reaching out to cover my hand with hers when I started crying. A mother without the heaviness of history. She continued to hold me in her gaze. "It can be scary not to have a diagnosis."

"Yes," I said, so thankful someone understood. So thankful to have the veil of acting fine lifted. I wiped at the tears dripping off my chin.

"Let's muscle test," she said. Half of me thought, What in the world? Where is the science behind that? And the other half of me thought, Who cares? She heard me when I talked. She can do whatever she wants.

I piled up mountains of hope on her thin shoulders.

She handed me test tubes, had me hold them up to my face one at a time and hold the other arm out parallel to the floor. She put two fingers on my wrist and pressed. Weirdly, sometimes I could resist the pressure and keep my arm where it was. Other times, it gave to her pressure. She looked at my tongue next.

"First of all," she said, "you should stop eating dairy."

No big loss. Ice cream gave me stomachaches, and creamy pasta dishes made me want to hurl. "Okay."

She had me lay on a table, tapped needles in everywhere, which strangely didn't hurt, and then left the room to mix up herbs. An overstuffed woman dancing around a moon hung directly overhead. She twisted slowly from the thread she hung from. I watched the pin in the ceiling instead because it was moving less. The room, along with the massage table I lay on, was afloat, sloshing and rocking erratically on a carpet sea. And then, out of nowhere, the sea calmed. My head cleared. The fog lifted and my brain returned to normal working order. I blinked into the blinding clarity of it. Without moving, I glanced from wall to wall. They were still. I wanted to scream, I wanted to jump up, run to find the acupuncturist and hug her tightly. Instead, one hot tear ran out of the corner of my eye, soaking the closest pin.

"It's working," I got out when the acupuncturist returned. "It's working," I whispered, checking the walls to make sure.

Next to the massage table, she tilted her head, smiled with what I assumed to be the burden of a world full of nonbelievers, and laid a hand on my shoulder. Patted a few times. "Good," she said simply.

But when she took the needles out, it all came rushing back in. Mad, it seemed, to have been displaced. I had to curl up on my side on the table and swallow spit, trying not to puke.

"It's alright," she said softly. "If it worked once, it will work again." I tucked her words into the back corner of my heart, repeated them over and over, a lifeline thrown just out of reach but swinging out there somewhere in the dark.

The acupuncturist fit me into her schedule for the following day and packed me off with powdery dirt to spoon into hot water and drink. I had to rest halfway down the short hallway in order to make it back outside.

I continued to see the acupuncturist twice a week because I could think clearly for the thirty minutes the needles were in. We identified the exact points at either temple that did the trick and called them the "dizzy drain." Each time, the minute the needles came out, the dizziness slammed back in, always kicked up and worse than before the needles. The heavy brain fog rolled back in on the heels of the dizziness. No matter what the acupuncturist tried, she couldn't get it to last after the needles were out. I kept handing over my credit card for the beauty of that thirty-minute break in which the sea stilled and the fog lifted and I could figure out what my next steps were going to be.

Mostly, what I thought about twice a week, as I stared at the overstuffed moon lady hanging from the ceiling, was whether or not the neurologist was a quack. The idea that a tumor might be growing in my brain day by day plagued me. The regular paychecks were enabling me to buy food and pay down the credit card little bit by little bit. An MRI would max it out. Which I was willing to do, if it seemed necessary. But my feet have always been ticklish. Maybe it was my ears, and the ENT I saw was wrong. Weren't there ENT tests? You can't see the inner ear by looking in. I would go back to the first ENT I saw, and this time, I would fight through the fog and the crushing motion of the overly lit room and assert myself.

■ ■ ■

A few weeks into dating, I showed up late to meet Mike for a movie. He'd been waiting twenty-five minutes. The movie had started. He was standing under a streetlamp out front as I bustled through the parking lot toward him, my heart pounding, my palms beginning to sweat.

"Sorry. I'm so sorry," I said as I walked up. "Are you mad?"

He tilted his head, hands in the pockets of his jeans, a grin spreading across his face like it always did when he saw me. "Why would I be mad?"

The clear night sky expanded infinitely behind him. Angry people had been a constant thrum in my life. His words crashed through me as unbelievable as a flash flood. He pulled me in close, and I rested my exhausted head against his chest. "Want to get something to eat instead? We can see the movie another time."

"You really aren't mad? I don't even have a good reason. You had to wait," I added as we walked to his truck. This couldn't last. But I wanted it to. Forever. I could hardly fathom a relationship with no dark corners, no false footing, no constant squaring off.

"Stop," he said, shaking his head, tightening his arm around my shoulders. "You were just late. It's no big deal. I'm hungry anyway. Where should we go?" He was the only place I could relax, let my guard down, rest. I wouldn't taint it with constant talk of dizziness and no money and doctors. I would confide in him, sure, but otherwise, I'd keep this one place as free of it as I could possibly manage.

■ ■ ■

I paid another $350 and sat in the airy lobby of the ENT's office. Eventually, I was shown into the small exam room. The only place for me to sit was in that stupidly reclined chair. I wanted to stand up, assert myself, but that's not what you do. You sit where you are supposed to. You show your most vulnerable parts to another human who doesn't in return. I perched on the edge of it. The first ENT I had seen back in January bustled into the room in the same flaring coattails kind of way, settled on the rolly seat with his back perfectly straight, and settled his eyes on me. "What can I do for you?"

This was a fantastic start. No computer sucking up his attention. Instead, he was focused on me. "I have some questions." I ignored the wall waterfall going on behind him. "How can we be sure it's not a problem with my inner ear? Isn't that usually the source of vertigo?"

He waggled his head. A jerky motion that caused the room to wobble even more than it already was. I squinted and tried to ignore the way I was slipping into its wobble.

"Not always," he said. "Could be cervical."

"The X-ray was normal," I countered. Now we were getting somewhere. Inching our way closer to that elusive middle ground between us. I readjusted on the edge of the annoying chair, ready to keep working at it, but he had turned away. His attention sucked up by the screen, his back to me.

"I'm prescribing PT for cervical vertigo," he said in a this-will-fix-it-I've-got-other-patients-waiting tone as he peered at the computer, filling in the right fields to make that happen. I wanted to say so much more. To ask if cervical vertigo shows up on X-rays or if I was in good company with others who had this diagnosis and clear X-rays, but he was done, and I had exhausted myself. Focusing enough to drive to his office had taken every ounce of energy I had. Focusing on the conversation had put me at a deficit, and his lack of interest had suddenly left me catatonic. How I was going to get home was the most pressing question I had, but I swallowed it along with all the others as he told me which way to turn to find my way out.

■ ■ ■

Several days later, after one of the two classes I was wasting unbelievable amounts of money on that semester, the physical therapist with the piercing sun slats led me back to the same exam room. I had to force myself over the threshold, dreading whatever she was going to do to me this time. Nothing had been explained to me except when and where to show up. I was not a person held underwater, caught in a net of fear. I was a body with a problem. I was no longer eligible for my university health insurance because I could not carry a full load of classes.

"Okay," the PT said, full of coffee and good cheer. She patted the exam table. "Go ahead and lay down."

I lay down carefully, trying to stall, to exert the last bit of control I had. She pulled her rolly chair up behind me where I couldn't see her. Her hands wrapped around my skull, making it feel small and insignificant. She probed at the small muscles and ran strong fingers deep into the larger ones. Tears leaked out of my eyes at the relief of it.

"Everything's locked up back here," she said. "You've probably been holding your head still to mitigate the dizziness."

Her hands, so violent before, kneaded steadily at the base of my skull, spreading a deep calm through every rigid inch of me. The brain fog lifted like those few extraordinary days a year when blue sky revealed itself over southeast Alaska. The ceiling above me still swayed but only vaguely. I blinked to make sure. This was it.

I have cervical vertigo, I told myself, settling into the relief of a correct diagnosis like a soft blanket just out of the dryer. *I have cervical vertigo*, I thought, *and all I need is a wonderful massage to make it go away. Or perhaps a series of massages. A massage every day.* I began to love the physical therapist, her strong hands that could clear storms.

As she continued the mind bending massage of whatever ball of muscle tucks into the back of the skull, life came back in little snippets of an imagined future: me participating in a conversation in a classroom at school, me at a computer working on my book, me up past 8:30 p.m., clinking my whiskey glass to Mike's. The magic massage worked the first couple times, holding off the dizziness for a number of hours before it showed up again, mad and raging. But by the third massage, the magic had worn off. The dizziness showed up before I made it back out to the parking lot. I dutifully continued to show up twice a week, filled with equal parts high, crushing hope that it might possibly work again and a hot, liquid dread that it would not.

After three months and an exploding credit card balance, I had to take off that comforting diagnosis and wander around again in the windy no man's land of wondering what could possibly be wrong with me.

The ENT shrugged, said, "Guess it's not cervical."

The PT didn't say much at all, just looked at me sadly.

If it wasn't my ears, it wasn't my eyes, and it wasn't cervical, then it had to be a brain tumor. And the fact that the dizziness was getting steadily worse was likely a sign that the tumor was growing. I set up a fifteen-minute phone call with the neurologist. Her receptionist explained to me that she billed fifty dollars per fifteen minutes for phone consultations. Desperate, I read off my credit card number and waited for her to call me back.

A few minutes later, the phone rang. I explained as quickly as possible, to keep out of the hundred-dollar range, how the dizziness had gotten worse since I'd seen her. How most nights I was curled up incapacitated by 6:30 p.m. "Do you still think it's a possibility I have a brain tumor? Do you think I need an MRI at this point?"

"Yes," she said. I wasn't sure if she'd answered yes to both questions or just the last one, and I couldn't muster the courage, or the energy, to ask. I'd flown to my mom's house for Christmas. The icy cold of the Michigan winter had seeped into me, had slowed me down even more. Or maybe it was the brain tumor.

I scheduled an MRI at the University of Michigan for the following day. My mom offered to pay for it, and shame crashed through me when I realized there was no way I could refuse. Since I'd left home with eighty dollars, Mom had helped when she could, but the reality was things were tight before the loss of my dad's income and extra tight afterward. Besides, I was almost thirty. I curled up on my childhood bed my dad had built and questioned every choice I had ever made. I should have dated men bound for Wall Street, not race car drivers and climbers and shipyard workers. I should have studied something practical like business in college, not field biology. I should have been putting money in a savings account instead of working on boats and flying around in bush planes.

The results of the MRI arrived a week later in a thin envelope mixed in with the rest of Mom's mail. My hand trembled as I held it. This was how I'd find out? Had someone really dropped a note in the mail that said, *Hey, sorry, it's a tumor*?

The possibility was so terrifying that I couldn't even open the envelope. I pressed my back against the wall in the hallway. How could the world possibly be so heartless to sick people? I knew the world was heartless, but this seemed beyond reason. Was human interaction too much to ask for? Were there too many humans? Too many people who come in for MRIs for a doctor or a technician or, hell, even a volunteer in a vest to make the celebratory phone call? *Hey! You're good! No tumors!* Or the opposite phone call? *I'm so sorry. I hear you. I understand. Here are the next steps to take.*

I peeled the envelope open and tried to catch the words as they slid around on the page.

The word "NORMAL" whipped past, and I crumpled to the floor.

■   ■   ■

By twenty-six years old, I had backpacked and camped and skied all over Colorado and Wyoming. I'd gotten lost, gotten frostbite, gotten myself through college, and currently had a job turning knobs in a loud, windowless chemistry lab in a subbasement.

Alaska seemed the next likeliest place to push at my edges, to live in that anything-can-happen-at-any-time place that I found necessary, to accumulate good stories to tell over campfires, to keep myself ready for the next roundhouse blow. I picked out the small cruise boat that I would want to be a passenger on if I could afford it. Since I couldn't, I applied for a job as a naturalist/kayak guide. I'd never been in a sea kayak before, so I told the guy I had good balance. For some reason, he hired me.

My job would be to answer questions passengers had about bears, whales, and glaciers. I'd never seen any of these things, so I memorized a thick binder of facts. There would be three real naturalists on board as well, so I planned to listen to them and soak it all up like a sponge while busying myself doing whatever else naturalist/kayak guides did besides answer questions.

The crew of fifteen met in Seattle for a bit of training while we got settled into the 150-foot powerboat. We left for Juneau a week later at dawn on a chilly, fog laden April morning.

That night, I woke up to the sound of crushing metal as I was thrown from my top bunk to the floor with the seven other women who'd been assigned bunks in the foc'sle.

It was pitch black, the seven of us were in a tangled pile, and everyone was screaming. I caught an elbow or knee in the lip and tasted blood before I caught another elbow or knee in the stomach. I launched out of the pile and was the first to the top of the stairs, out of the bow, and up onto the main floor.

The engineer ran past in sweatpants and no shirt, his face tight, yelling into his radio, "We're taking on water!"

The boat continued its slow tilt to starboard until the wooden bar and bolted down stools were at a forty-five-degree angle.

I clung to a bolted table in the dining room, my stomach seizing as I imagined the boat going down, me trapped inside, water filling my lungs, the heaviness of it.

In the middle of the roll back the other direction, I sprinted across the common area to the stairs at the stern. I needed to be outside, up above, where I could swim away instead of getting trapped underneath. I arrived on the top deck, as wild as the storm we were caught in and out of breath. The sea was an angry mixture of whipping rain and chaotic waves. Several crew members huddled next to the life raft, wearing bright orange horse-collar life jackets. Someone shoved one at me, and I pulled it over my head and cinched it up tight around my chest. My T-shirt and thin shorts soaked through as the rain slashed against me sideways.

One of the deckhands stood ready to launch the bright orange lifeboat at the captain's word. The second mate ran toward us through the rain, the wind rippling his clothes. He had on glasses rather than his usual contacts, jeans and a T-shirt rather than his usual perfectly ironed uniform. His feet were bare and pale against the dark night.

"Now?" the deckhand yelled as the boat began its roll toward the side where we were standing. His hand gripped the release for the lifeboat. No one spoke as the water got closer and closer to the railing, green and foamy.

"Not yet," the second mate said, his face drawn and gray. "Coast Guard's on its way." The thump of the helicopter was somewhere in the dark of the sky beyond the mountainous waves. "We're stuck on a rock. Better if we can get loose before we launch lifeboats." He grabbed another deckhand's shoulder. "Get everyone out and up here, ready to go," he shouted and then turned, clawing back toward the pilothouse along the railing.

We all hung on as the boat rolled back to flat and then up onto the opposite side. The deck fell away into a sheer drop-off to the sea below, and my mind emptied of everything else aside from the knowledge that I would soon be in the cold, tossing water. Dad was close. He always was when situations began to spin wildly out of control. Some faded out version of him was ahead of me on this path, looking back, nodding, his face bright, as if to say, *Now you're in the shit! Let's see you shine!* I leaned into his half presence, into the pressing clarity of crisis, and found what he'd been offering all along. A deep well of resilience. If I ended up in the water, alright. If I didn't, alright. Fear evaporated and an eerie calm spread through me.

The engines gunned in reverse as we swung through the trough of the next roll. The boat shook violently under my feet in response. Another four crew members hustled up the back stairs in a tight group, with the deckhand on their heels. One was crying, the other three were eerily quiet. The deckhand tossed life jackets at them, and one of the bartenders went around tightening the chest straps on everyone.

The frantic roaring of the engine shuddered through my body. The boat seemed to be coming apart until, with a hard lurch that tossed us all, it finally ripped free of the rock.

I held my breath, trying to figure out if we were actually sinking now. Wouldn't it be so slow that you wouldn't realize it at first? The water continued to whip and fling itself all around us as the helicopter ran its spotlight from bow to stern, apparently trying to figure out the same thing. My teeth clacked together uncontrollably as the cold and rain entered my bones.

The second mate showed up again to explain that we weren't taking on water, that the waves had been strong enough to bust through the watertight seal on the stern door, drenching the engine room in salt water. He herded everyone back into the main dining area of the boat, where we could get to the lifeboats in a hurry if necessary. I was full body shivering but stayed out at the rail with the wispy traces of my dad, rain driving at my face, running down my neck.

The helicopter peeled off into the night when a Canadian Coast Guard boat showed up to escort us to the nearest Canadian harbor, and Dad faded into the night.

When my legs went numb, I went inside. The crew had turned into unmoving, dark lumps in the dining room. There was a movie playing, but no one was watching it. It was 4:00 a.m., but no one was going back to bed. We were two hours away from the nearest dock. Everyone seemed to be watching and waiting. I changed into dry clothes and joined the head chef and sous chef on a bench seat next to a big, cold window.

"Did you hear?" the sous chef asked. His hair was flung out in all directions and was still damp from the rain. "The captain and third mate are drunk. We were miles off course."

"Where are they now?" I asked, realizing neither were in the dining room, imagining them bound and gagged somewhere in the depths of the ship.

"In their quarters." His face set, hard. "Probably so we don't rip them to shreds."

A small pack of Canadian Coast Guard men in sharp uniforms were waiting for us at 6:00 a.m. as we eased up to the dock. The captain and third mate were escorted off the boat in handcuffs, and most of the crew, including every naturalist but me, quit.

The following day, a shiny new captain flew in from Seattle and limped the boat up to Ketchikan to the nearest dry dock, where it was hauled out to fix the damage to the hull.

With the boat towering over me, I walked underneath the bulbous bow, a two-foot-by-four-foot chunk of concrete encased metal that the impact had completely crushed. I stared at the wreckage, calculating the distance from where my head had been laying on my pillow to the point of direct impact: maybe five feet.

In the bare bones trip up to Ketchikan, the second mate had explained to me that very few boats have bulbous bows. It was an awkward feature sometimes added to boats to create better stability in the Caribbean, which is where our particular boat had come from. "Without that ugly piece of concrete up there," the second mate had gone on to say, "the impact would've ripped a six-foot hole in the hull." Right through my bunk.

After a week in dry dock, we arrived in Juneau to pick up our first load of passengers, with me as the only naturalist on board.

As we snaked our way through huge icebergs dotted with hauled-out harbor seals, killer whales swimming off in the distance, mountains rising straight up from the water's edge, I stood on the deck, mesmerized by this place I'd almost not made it to. The strength and power of so much undisturbed land pulled at me until the edges of me dissolved into the edges of it. With the mixing, I felt stronger and more solid than I could ever feel on my own. I stood among the passengers on the deck, half terrified someone would ask me a question I didn't know the answer to and half not caring because the breeze off the glacier at the end of the fjord had just reached us. In my binder of facts, I'd read this was common. Wind often rolled down the steep slope of a glacier and blew steadily through the adjoining fjord.

I turned my face to it, closed my eyes. There is an old family story about how I cried more than I slept in my first year of life. My parents read the books, asked the doctor, tried everything. Nothing worked until, in a moment of desperation, my father carried me out onto the second story deck of the cabin where we lived in Northern Michigan and held me up to the wind, which calmed my cries that night, and all the rest of the nights that the wind blew.

The long arms of the glacial breeze wrapped around me, and that part of me that had been silently crying for years began to settle.

■ ■ ■

The dizziness steadily increased over the few days following the normal MRI news, until I lay curled up on my side, afraid to move any part of my body because the minute I moved, the world would spin out of control. The jail cell got colder and danker, the toilet in the corner nastier. I was filled with anxiety so high I began to pretend I was someone else. I was an old man (I don't know why) from England (even weirder) with a gentle wife and grown children. A man prone to thin sweaters, laughing with his whole body, watching birds at his many feeders. He'd struggled through his life, celebrated plenty, and knew it was now coming to a close. I spent hours basking in the sweet relief of a life in which the end was in sight.

My mom knew a good neurologist at the University of Michigan who made room for me on his schedule. I white-knuckled the passenger seat as the car bucked and rolled across town to his office. He was a nice, older, efficient man with a gray mustache. I tried to focus, to make the most out of the allotted time, but I was consumed with trying to stay upright as the room boiled around me. My brain had turned to gelatin so that when I tried to explain what had been happening, I forgot parts, and my sentences drifted off into incoherence.

"Sounds like a vestibular migraine," he said after I got lost in a series of incomplete sentences. Had I said something about a headache? But he'd turned to his computer, had become a hunched back in a clean white coat. I didn't have a headache. Not the kind I'd heard about, where you need a dark room and no noise. Although I did hate noise. You don't move to the middle of nowhere Alaska if you are a person who likes noise. I'd always been the one to turn the radio down a notch on a fun Friday night, the one who got tired of the club first.

I didn't have a migraine. Just as I was about to explain that there was no headache or swirling colors, he said, "I'm going to prescribe Topamax." He was still tapping at the keys, back to me. A drug that could fix this flickered a small flare of hope, like a finally located lighter in the bottom of a pack on a cold, rainy camping trip. That rare blade of hope made me forget any other questions I might've asked. "You'll need to take it for three months to see if it works. If you stop early, we'll never know."

I knew he'd come to a hasty decision based on the crap intel I'd handed over. I needed more time to find the words to explain the intricacies of sick land so that he could think through the possibilities that existed over there in healthy doctor land, but he was up and moving toward the door. And then he was gone.

I dropped my head into my hands in the quiet room. Maybe he was right. He's a doctor. He knows more than I do.

Mom drove us straight to the pharmacy from the doctor's office. I ignored what he said about three months and instead imagined swallowing a pill, waking up the next day to a still room. I almost cried with relief, but the ability to cry was buried under the weight of existing in this minute and the next and the next in an endless forever. I wanted the pill to be big and white and chalky. The kind that were terrible going down because they were so necessary to so many, there was no time to dye them a pleasing orange and add a sugar coating. No time to stamp the company name on each individual capsule. They were so needed, so important, that they flew out of the factory in their raw glory.

When it was my turn at the pharmacy, the woman behind the counter said, "Insurance card?" after I gave her my name and date of birth.

"I don't have one."

She flicked her gaze up at me.

"I have a job. I'm just here for Christmas. It hasn't turned into full-time work yet. It's a preexisting condition." Why could I babble now and not in the sterile room with the cold doctor in a starched coat? I felt suddenly certain that I did not have a migraine. Who has a migraine without a headache? Why didn't I ask that? The woman bagged up a one-month supply of the prescription, slid it toward me, and said, "That'll be $400." "Without insurance," she added.

It's a broken system! I wanted to yell at the smug woman in the snappy blue pharmacy vest. *Just wait,* I wanted to say, *until you get sick one day and no one gives a fuck.* Instead, I handed over my credit card.

I broke into the packaging the minute I was back in the passenger seat. "What's wrong?" asked Mom.

"It's orange."

She gave me a worried look and then started the car.

I swallowed the pill dry, letting it scratch on the way down.

The next morning, I was worse.

The morning after that, I had an overwhelming sense that nothing mattered. I tried to be the English guy again, but I didn't care about him anymore. The next day, I was going to have to achieve the monumental task of getting myself on a plane back to Colorado.

I forced myself to go for a walk in the woods around my mom's house. Being outside always fueled me, and I needed fuel. The snow crunched under my feet. The single digit morning stung in my lungs in a way I typically liked but couldn't get myself to on that particular morning. The way the snow piled up on the boughs of conifers and on the ground up to my knees when I cut off the path should've cheered me. *The creek,* I thought. *The sound of the small creek will surely crack through the dark, heavy fields of depression.*

As I got close, I heard the small sound of water running under ice. I wanted to sit at its bank, let the natural world work its magic on me. With a gloved hand, I pushed aside a branch heavy with snow, and there at my feet was a fawn, curled up tight. Frozen solid. A light dusting of snow had gathered on its freckled back. Its eyes were closed, its face relaxed in sleep, the creek bubbling just beyond. I sat with the deer a long time. Took in the tucked-up legs, the rounded back, the tilt of its head resting on a pillow of snow. It was the perfect response to such a brutal world. To curl up in a beautiful place, close your eyes, let the cold turn to misperceived warmth, and fall asleep forever.

YEAR TWO

CHAPTER FIVE

Over the next few weeks, the world continued to pound and crash around me. The dizziness was so much worse for no apparent reason. The guy who supervised the lab quit; I took over all his shifts and the scheduling and became full time with benefits. If I could actually make it through forty hours of work a week, the preexisting condition clause would be met in six months' time and doctors would suddenly cost me the price of a pizza. Six months stretched into an eternity, but I forced myself not to think about it.

Every day was the same: I knew I couldn't make it through work, I decided I had to make it through work, I stayed at work.

On my days off, I fumbled through whatever had to be done that day and curled up in bed around 6:00 p.m. and thought about snow laden trees, the creek running by, the fawn curled up tight, the light dusting of snow on its back.

I dropped the few writing classes I had so hopefully enrolled in, stopped working on my novel. My brother started calling more often. Mike's face creased with a permanent worry.

A dark, growing force inside me, the dizziness developed the ability to, once or twice a day, throw me hard to the ground. I would grasp at whatever was close by—a table, a wall, a person—desperate to not hit the ground with such force. I did not fall toward the ground. I was never falling toward the ground. It was all in my head. I began to wonder if it was psychosomatic. If I was hysterical. Maybe I could stop it if only I could concentrate hard enough. Or maybe I needed a therapist and antidepressants. But who wouldn't be depressed if they'd been seasick for a year? I wasn't depressed when it started. Or maybe that's like an alcoholic who swears up and down it's not a problem.

Just shy of the one-month mark of Topamax, I called the neurologist's office at the University of Michigan. The receptionist connected me to his PA, who answered the phone cheerily enough.

"Yeah, hi. I'm wondering if the doctor could talk to my neurologist here in Colorado?" I asked. It seemed like a good idea to have the guy in Michigan discuss his ideas about vestibular migraine with the doctor in Colorado so she could take it from there.

The PA's voice turned to tacks. "You have a neurologist in Colorado?"

The river floor moved beneath me. I closed one eye to slow it down. "Yes. If they could talk, it would be helpful. She's not come to the same conclusion as he has, although the Topamax doesn't seem to be doing anything for the dizziness, and I can't stop thinking about, well, dead deer. If he could explain to her why he came to that diagnosis, she could continue my care here, where I live, and I could maybe ask a few follow-up questions now that I'm a month into the new medication and am not sure I can handle it for another two months. Unless the doctor there is available for a follow-up over the phone?"

"Why are you seeing two neurologists?" she asked sharply.

The story was so long, and I was so tired. The silence stretched as I tried to figure out where to start. Because a weird woman tickled my foot and I'm worried she doesn't have common sense? Because every day, dizziness is a slick, desperate place that leads to rash decisions? It was almost impossible to think through the Topamax brain cobweb that had settled on top of the dizziness brain fog.

"This is a pattern exhibited by drug seekers," she said.

I blinked. Suddenly, there were so many things to say. The first being, Who the fuck would want Topamax? I mean, maybe Valium or something with street value to help pay for these fucking doctors. But Topamax?

"Hello?" she said, impatient now.

But there were too many boundaries between us: sick/ healthy, patient/provider, broke/probably not broke, not able to think/able to think, powerful/weak. Impossible to get through. What would happen when I asked for my records to be sent to some future doctor and there was a note in there about me being a drug seeker? I needed these people. If I added even one more barrier between myself and them, I would be on my own forever.

"Hello," she said again, taking my silence for an admission of guilt or a stalling tactic perhaps.

I hung up the phone, curled up on the couch like the deer, imagined snow falling, the sound of the creek, the way cold turns warm if you're out in it too long.

■   ■   ■

The Michigan neurologist never followed up with the foot tickler or me to switch my prescription. The first month's prescription of the Topamax ran out. It wasn't making even the smallest bit of difference in the dizziness. If anything, it seemed to be making it worse, and the suicidal thoughts were terrifying me.

I wasn't living. I was just surviving. I couldn't hike or bike or run. I couldn't ski, I couldn't read, I couldn't be any type of partner Mike deserved. I wasn't fun. I had no idea why he didn't call it off and tried to prepare myself for the day he would.

I spent all my energy making it through eight hours of work in order to pay my credit card bill and get to that magic mark where insurance would start paying for doctors. I didn't have a headache or an aura or anything else associated with migraine. His diagnosis had to be wrong. All I knew for sure was that it was dangerous to stay in the dark place the drug had dropped me. I considered calling his office again, trying to talk to him this time to ask him if I should keep going, if the depression and cobweb head was normal, if both cleared out eventually for most people. I wanted to ask him what he might suggest next, but I didn't want to talk to the finger pointing PA again. And besides, obviously, when you called the doctor's office and asked to speak to the doctor, the answer was going to be a hard no.

Even worse than the dark Topamax place was the dark no-diagnosis, this-may-go-on-forever place.

I forced myself back to the Google. In three-minute computer intervals across many days, I found an ENT who specialized in dizziness. Maybe the first two I saw weren't specialized enough to figure out a complex problem. I called the office and asked how much it would cost to see the doctor without insurance.

"Eight hundred dollars," the receptionist said politely.

I pulled the phone away from my ear to hit the red hang-up button, but my thumb stalled out. Did it really matter if my credit card bill was five digits when I died face down in the dirt at forty-five? Probably not.

"Hello?" the woman said.

I slowly raised the phone back to my ear. "Okay," I said. "That's fine." Some small part of me that was still intact despite the dizziness wanted to laugh. How could that possibly be fine?

"Her next available is two months from tomorrow."

I made the appointment, hung up the phone, and dropped my head to the cold, hard wood of the table, trying to imagine surviving another two months before someone had the time to help me.

The next day, I was consumed with the idea that if I could just endure two more black months, maybe the Topamax would flip some sort of switch, and the door of the jail cell would magically open. Maybe that's how Topamax works. I'd never taken a drug long term before. Maybe the day it starts to work comes out of nowhere. I wanted to ask the doctor, but navigating the PA felt like too much to handle.

■ ■ ■

Two months later, the world was a hazy, hateful place. I hadn't worked on my novel in months, had barely eaten, and the dizziness continued to rage. My ears began to ring so loudly it was often hard to hear. There had been no "Hey, you okay?" check-in from the Michigan neurologist. Obviously. That blade of hope that it might be vestibular migraine and that Topamax would hand me myself back turned sharp and cut to the bone.

The $800 doctor was young, her hair bobbed. She looked me over as I perched on the edge of the exam table, white-knuckling it. She turned her back in the usual way and began filling in narrow computer fields. I glanced at the screen and felt a burst of hatred for all things bright and flashy. I answered her questions about Grandma, Grandpa, Mom, Dad, the elbow surgery in 1985 in a monotone, trying to save my energy for the real conversation.

She took me out into the hallway and asked me to walk a straight line. She walked along beside me with a hand at my back, likely because it was already clear it wasn't going to go well. She guided me back toward her just before I walked into the wall. She asked me to stand on one foot and caught me before I realized I was falling.

She led me back into the small exam room. "It's not vestibular," she said, helping me sit down again on the crinkly paper that now stuck to my sweaty hands. "It's structural," she added.

I waited for her to tell me what to do next. She did not.

"Who do I see for that?"

She lifted one shoulder. "That's outside my realm of expertise."

"A chiropractor?" I pressed. "A spine doctor? There was nothing wrong with the X-ray of my spine." I wondered suddenly if whoever read it, read it correctly. Are these people to be trusted? What if the X-ray reader had the end-all-be-all fight of his marriage right before getting to work and missed something minute? Perhaps an X-ray reader at a major hospital would catch some small abnormality that a student health center guy would miss? Was that a shitty thing to think?

"What do you think?" I asked the doctor.

She waggled her head noncommittally. "It's not a problem with your ears."

Wasn't there some sort of overview in medical school? Some sort of flowchart: if it's not this, it might be this? And besides, she was the one with the brain that worked. I took a deep breath. Tried so hard to say, *Please help.* The words tunneling up from that deep, dark place there seemed to be no way out of.

But I was too slow, the words buried under too much rubble. She was standing up, and I was too. I gathered up my coat, and she followed me out into the hallway. She walked next to me, her hand on my lower back again as I headed to the front desk to hand my card over. To pay almost a thousand dollars for a shrug. I tried to feel grateful—she was obviously worried I'd walk into the wall again—but I couldn't even look at her. She bent down to the receptionist and said something I couldn't hear over the noise in my head.

The receptionist nodded, tapped twice at her computer, and held out her hand for my credit card. "That'll be one hundred dollars."

The doctor straightened up and caught my eye. In her look, I saw that she had actually seen me. She had heard what I was not saying. That I was at the end of my rope in every way possible: physically, emotionally, financially.

I tried again to feel grateful that she had miraculously lowered her rate to something reasonable, but that shrug played over and over in my mind. I wanted to shrug back now that it was my turn. But I couldn't. "Thank you," I said, dropping my eyes, taking my place below her in the animal kingdom of the health care system: patient/doctor, broke/not broke, weak/powerful.

■ ■ ■

I clawed my way back into the world of my novel. I lived on boats and fished in the rain as often as I could. I numbered the handwritten pages and slid them into a blue folder. Pages and pages and pages piled up. A series of slanted, chicken scratched lines saving me night after night in the dim clickety clack of the lab.

"I can help," Mike said, pointing at the blue folder one afternoon as I stuffed it into my bag on my way to work. "I'm good at typing."

I froze. "You'd do that for me?"

"Were you planning to send it out to agents like that?" He pointed again at the folder in my hand.

"I'd stand out at least."

"Like some crotchety old grandma who refused to learn email. Hand it over."

"The crotchety part is right."

He reached out a hand for the folder, and instead, I sagged into his arms. "And I may have to give up email."

That night, and for a lot of nights to come, while I scrawled away at work, he sat in the blue recliner at home and deciphered the second most vulnerable way I lived in the world.

■ ■ ■

Chiropractors are less expensive than out-of-pocket spine doctors, so I started there.

The first chiropractor was a big man, his hands at his sides like coiled snakes when he walked into the exam room. I sat in a hard plastic chair against the wall, weary of the exam table.

"Alright," he said with very white teeth as he settled himself in front of the computer. He asked some questions I answered while appreciating the dimness of the room. The small lamp on a small table. He seized on the gymnastics in my past.

"Any big falls?" he asked.

"Yes."

"Hmmm," he said, as if the puzzle pieces were falling into place. "C'mon up." He patted the exam table.

I lay down, anxiety swallowing me. I wanted to be able to see him. To anticipate. If he made the dizziness worse, I wasn't sure I would survive it. His hands cupped my entire head in the way mine cup a coffee mug. He began to probe the area where my spine connects to my skull. *Be careful*, I wanted to say.

"Hmm . . ." he said again.

"What?" I said, taut as a piano string.

"There's pressure here between C1 and the occipital. A common cause for dizziness."

Hope is a dangerous thing. It swells like a helium balloon in the chest, lifting you out of whatever hellish situation you are in. It floats you through the perfect blue sky, the Earth rolling out below you with all of its imperfections blurring into a beautiful geometric pattern below. The sun is warm on your back, you are light as air until hope bursts and you are in free fall, the unforgiving cracked dirt coming fast enough to explode bones.

"I'm going to need you to relax as best you can while I do the adjustment," he said. As he got to his feet, hovered over me like a runner about to sprint, and wrapped his huge hands around my head, my heart raced, and I broke out in a cold sweat. He felt me ready to fight him and said, "Relax. You can trust me," before he did something so violent with my head that adrenaline colored everything in reds and blues. I lay panting as his fingers prodded the back of my neck. I focused on the ceiling, breathing into my ramming heart, like someone staring at the sky from the pavement after a car wreck. My mind raced, trying to get a handle on the new situation. Is it worse? Is it worse? Am I okay?

As the adrenaline drained out, so did the dizziness.

He finished prodding the base of my skull and said, "That should be better." And it was.

I sat up. He no longer looked big. His hands just looked like hands. He smiled, and I decided I was all wrong. He was a really nice man.

"Thank you," I said, checking the walls, the carpet, for movement. They both still moved and slid but not as much.

"We'll see you in a few days, then. Have Debbie get you on the schedule for twice a week for the next few weeks. We'll get you fixed right up."

He left, and I slid back into my shoes, put my earrings back in, the balloon full, lifting me up. It was structural. There would be no other horrible drugs. Hands would fix me. I would finish school, finish the novel, be what Mike deserved, make friends.

■ ■ ■

It was the breathing that woke me up.

A series of short sniffs in and then a forced exhalation through the nose. The pale Alaskan morning light was diffused even further by the blue fabric of my tent. I lifted my head slowly to look through the mesh zippered door and met the eyes of a brown bear.

His next exhalation blew the hair off my forehead.

My first week off the cruise ship lined up with one of the deckhand's, so we'd teamed up for a five-day kayaking trip. It's much safer to paddle with another person in the backcountry, unless of course that person is the particular deckhand who was available for me to paddle with.

While I brought canned beans, apples, and tortillas, he brought a five-day supply of Snickers bars for breakfast, lunch, and dinner. Even though I'd asked him three times, I was fairly certain he'd had one on him when he'd climbed into the tent the night before.

The deckhand hadn't brought a tent to Alaska, so he was sharing mine.

The bear pressed his massive head against the mesh fabric of the tent door, his eyes rolling over the contents of the tent. Spiders of fear skittered through my body, both freezing me in place and clearing my mind in the way only moments like this can. It was his move. He snorted and turned abruptly. His stomach sagged toward the ground, the shaggy brown side of him as big as a mattress. I forced air into my lungs and unzipped the tent as noiselessly as possible. I peeked around the edge of the tent. The bear had lumbered over to our double kayak and was pushing it toward the water with his head. I dropped back inside, slapped at the still sleeping deckhand, and shoved both feet into boots. "Get up!" I whisper yelled.

If the bear got the kayak to the water, the outgoing tide would carry it swiftly out of the bay and down the channel. There would be no swimming for it in the frigid water that makes your legs and arms stop working after seven minutes. We would miss the boat pickup, a six-hour paddle away. If we didn't show up, it would take them days, possibly weeks, to search the quadrant of the 3.3-million-acre park we had indicated we'd be paddling in. We had one day of food left. This was long before cell phones worked in southeast Alaska, and who had the money for a sat phone? Not us.

The deckhand woke with a start. He stared at me through squinted eyes and California tanned hair. He sat up at the sound of the kayak rolling over on the rocks. "Bear," I whispered, now crouching in the vestibule of the tent, keeping out of sight of the bear. The deckhand kicked out of his sleeping bag and scrambled to pull on boots. "He's almost got the kayak to the water."

"We'll hold the sleeping bag between us to look bigger and make a run for it," he speed whispered, pushing up to a crouch in the vestibule.

"Don't run. He'll chase," I said.

"I can outrun him," he said, gathering up the sleeping bag. The deckhand was twenty-two years old.

"No. You. Can't," I hissed, ducking back in for the can of bear spray in the side pocket of the tent.

The bear continued to push the kayak with his head until it was ten feet from the water's edge, at which point, my bright yellow dry bag tumbled free. It contained the clothes I cooked in, which I kept separate from the clothes I slept in. We watched, still crouched in the vestibule, peeking over the top of the tent in the dull morning light as the bear abandoned the kayak and pounced on the dry bag like a cat, front paws out, back end high up in the air. One of his three-inch claws easily sliced through the tough vinyl.

The bear collapsed his massive furry back end onto the beach, got a better grip on the dry bag with his two front paws, and then used the smallest of his front teeth to tug gently at the layers of wool, Carhartt, and sweatshirt now exposed. He extracted my bra by its strap until the rest of it got caught in the narrow rip of the dry bag. He yanked harder. When this didn't work, he readjusted his bite on the strap and then whipped his head hard to the left. The bra snagged up one more time on the dry bag, then ripped free with enough momentum to wap him in the face.

"What the hell," the deckhand breathed out.

The bear pinned the offending undergarment to the small, dark rocks of the beach with a dinner plate sized paw and fixed his gaze on us.

"That's gonna be gross to put back on," the deckhand said.

The bear pounced again on the dry bag and this time yanked out one leg of my Carhartts. He ran like a puppy with the pant leg in his mouth and flung the bag up in the air and pounced again.

"This is not the kind of shit they show on the Discovery Channel." The deckhand stared as the bear flung and pounced again.

The bear looked up. Abandoned the dry bag, took a few running steps toward us. We jumped up from our crouched position behind the tent and snapped the sleeping bag taut between us to look as big as possible. I slid the safety off the bear spray. The bear became distracted by some scent, swung his massive head away to look toward the woods in the opposite direction.

We took a couple quiet, tentative steps before the bear turned back and sprinted all out, straight at us.

"Ahhh!" the deckhand yelled.

We dropped the sleeping bag, hauled ass to the kayak, smacked and splashed our way in, and paddled hard. Bears can swim, but this one, for whatever reason, decided not to.

As we glided across the smooth water, breathing hard, the bear loping off in the opposite direction, I decided I'd do whatever it took to stay in a place so unabashedly truthful about how life and death are an equal possibility in every moment. Of course, we all know this, but in cities, in the suburbs, we wrap ourselves in the idea that the two are distinct. But after my dad was there one minute and gone the next, I constantly wanted to shake people and say, *Don't you see?* I wanted to live in a place that externally matched what I knew to be true internally. And I had found it.

■ ■ ■

When I moved into Mike's house, everything I owned fit in my car. It took about an hour to add my books to the bookshelf, put my unused skis in the basement, tuck my socks next to his in the sock drawer.

Mike's solid presence, his quiet house, and the way his dog liked to put his head in my lap took the edge off the endless days. I didn't talk to Mike much about the dizziness. Or at least not much compared to how it rodeoed around my thoughts at all times. I never told him about the fawn. I wanted him to be in a relationship with me, not me and my illness. I didn't really pull this off. He was certainly in a relationship with me and my illness, but I tried to hold back the worst of it. He deserved so much better.

"I love you," I said every day because I didn't know how to say all the rest of it.

"I love you," he said back. There was no if-only-you'd-act-this-way, there was no I-need-you-to . . . There were no minefields to creep through, no imminent volcano of anger slowly burbling. I had no idea it could be so simple, so straightforward, so well lit. And I didn't want to lose it.

I continued to see the chiropractor twice a week for months. It turned violent. Sometimes he made the dizziness better, and sometimes he made it dramatically worse. When he made it better, it would only last a few hours. When he made it worse, it would last weeks. I began to hate the submissive act of lying down, that he attacked from outside my field of vision.

I felt more settled that the problem was structural and that this particular chiropractor could not get a handle on it, but I felt the need to check in with the nurse practitioner. I needed a partner in crime. Someone to work together to hash out probabilities, to formulate plans L and M and N. If there were options, there was hope. Eight chiropractic appointments a month weren't cheap, but if we decided together that it made sense, then I'd keep at it.

A week later, the nurse practitioner leaned forward on the rolly seat as I sat on the sticky paper.

"If it's not a problem with my ears, my eyes, or a brain tumor, it's got to be structural right?" I asked. "Unless the muscle tightness and pressure between C1 and the occipital are just a result of being dizzy for a year. I hold my head really still. Makes sense that everything would tighten up."

She squinted. "I'm not convinced it's structural. If it was, then the chiropractic work shouldn't have such a varied outcome."

"Exactly," I said, afraid of letting go the comfortable sweater of a diagnosis but feeling the first strands of hope that the next one might fit better.

"Have you been taking the CoQ10?"

"Yes."

"Does it help?"

"No."

"And the ENTs have said it's not your ears, correct?"

"Correct."

She spun to her desk and began writing something down. "It's time for you to go see a friend of mine. She's a bodyworker." She handed me a piece of paper with a name and a number.

"What's a bodyworker do?" I asked. I didn't want a bodyworker. I wanted a scientific direction. I wanted an answer.

"Miracles."

CHAPTER SIX

I sat in my car outside the bodyworker's office for a long time, thinking of all the reasons I didn't want to walk in. But desperation had been gagging up my throat so bad lately, I stuffed my wallet and keys in my jeans pocket and crossed the street to her front door.

Her office was in a historic house with creaky floors in a suburb of Denver. A receptionist sat at a small square table with nothing on it but a computer. The living room turned waiting area was decorated with a few fashion-over-function, mustard colored chairs. The receptionist brightly explained they took cash or check or card. I watched her slide my card through that narrow slot on the side that my eyes and hands would not have been able to line up. I watched her hair fall over her shoulder, the ease in her slim form suggesting she could do anything she wanted.

Once my signature was vaguely on the line it was supposed to be on, she led me to a bedroom turned exam room. "Go ahead and lie down," she said, gently tapping the padded table as if it were normal to submit, even if you didn't know what was coming. At least there was a sheet and not the sticky paper. I sat on the edge of the exam table.

The bodyworker had flyaway hair and ruddy skin, no makeup. "Sandy called me and told me all about what's going on," she said as she walked in. "I'm so sorry this has been going on for so long for you."

It threw me at first, the nurse practitioner's first name, but then I began to feel like perhaps I had been let into a sisterhood of healing. Like there was a genuine interest that would lead to a genuine result. I lay down when she asked me to. She took four deep breaths, and then, with her eyes half closed, she began to run her hands over my body, leaving a couple inches between her hands and my chest, my arms, my legs, my head. If I couldn't understand the dizziness, why did I need to understand the treatment? I relaxed, let her do whatever she was doing, felt the balloon filling, began to rise above the mess of it all.

Her eyes still closed, her hands still moving, she said, "You have a brother."

I tried to recall if I'd told the nurse practitioner I had a brother. I didn't think so.

"You have spent previous lifetimes together," she went on. "Your parents were killed, and the two of you hid from the Germans in the war-torn streets of Europe. As the eldest, you were responsible for him. You are still carrying this fear."

For fuck's sake.

The balloon popped, and I slammed into the ground, hard, arms out to brace the fall, but no luck, my face slammed into the dirt.

She opened her eyes, dropped her hands, and smiled.

She had me sit up slowly, possibly because I looked so shaken. She disappeared down the hall on silent feet and then came back with a small vial of brown pellets that I was to swallow four times a day for a week.

Desperation turned to shame as I sat in a restaurant over a lunch I couldn't eat and shook out five small, hard, brown pellets. I swallowed them down, rationalizing that I did, actually, have a lot of fear, that the dizziness felt as dangerous as the Germans.

■ ■ ■

"You okay?" Mike asked one night over dinner.

"Yeah," I answered automatically.

He reached across the table for my hand.

"Not really," I corrected. But how to say all the rest? Time itself bends into something unrecognizable when you live with chronic illness. 'Live in the moment', all those well-hydrated people say, but fuck, it would be nice to make plans for lunch with a friend the following day and not worry over if you'll be able to actually function tomorrow at noon. It would be nice to imagine a future of some sort that wasn't about surviving one minute and fearing the onset of the next because it might be worse. When health, all of the future, and health care itself have become a privilege not available to you, how do you answer the question: 'Are you okay?'

As the silence stretched and that line between sick/not sick bolded itself between us, Mike squeezed my hand and said gently, "How about a therapist?"

"Depression doesn't cause dizziness," I shot back. Not Mike too.

"Right," he said gently. "But dizziness causes depression."

■ ■ ■

I found a therapist close to home. She wore a swishy skirt as she led me to a room at the end of a hallway. A sandbox stood in the corner, which was a little worrisome.

It felt good to talk, at first.

I showed up every two weeks, as the therapist suggested. The only really great thing was how much less stressed Mike looked.

What was there to work through? To get to the bottom of? It was simple: I was stuck on the crumbling shoulder of life, I wanted back out onto the paved lanes of traffic with everyone else, but I wasn't allowed out there because I had a shitty, broken-down car, and I was depressed because of it. There was no solution to find through talking. *Expect this*, my dad had said. *And you'll be able to handle it.* Except I wasn't handling it. And could he even have fathomed this? It was worse than having a broken-down boat car. It was like having a broken-down bicycle. And no legs.

The only solution lay in gritting my teeth, bearing the weight of every day until my insurance would allow me to see as many doctors as I needed at whatever insane price they charged, until I found one who could help. My body worked right for thirty-one years, surely there was a path back to it. And if there wasn't any help to be had, I would curl up next to a creek on a snowy day and give in.

"What can we do to help you find a way to live with this?" the therapist asked, her long, stringy hair poking the tops of her thighs as she leaned forward in her chair.

Live with it? The world sloshing and tossing me about, nauseous and exhausted and unable to think forever?

She changed tack when she noticed the horrified expression. It took so much energy to talk, and I still had to drive home, get myself to work, stay there for eight hours somehow. "What do you miss most?" she asked.

"Books." I tried every few weeks to see if I could magically, suddenly read again, but after a few pages, words slipped and slid, my stomach lurched as if I were on a roller coaster, and I'd have to close my eyes and ride out the imagined-but-real Space Mountain. I had spent a lifetime finding refuge in books, and for the first time ever, there was nowhere to go.

"I can fill out paperwork to give you access to the Library for the Blind," the therapist said. Her face was perfectly round and constantly flushed.

"I'm going to learn braille?" I imagined an unrecognizable version of myself reading with my hands.

"They have audiobooks. You don't have to be blind to qualify. They also serve the visually handicapped."

She placed the word around my neck like a lei, as if I had just arrived in Hawaii. It hung heavy against my chest.

"They have an enormous selection," she was saying. "Much bigger than any public library."

I'd thought about getting audiobooks from the library, but in the past, when I'd looked for a book to listen to for various road trips, I'd always had a hard time finding anything I was all that interested in.

■ ■ ■

A man named Dennis answered the phone at the Library for the Blind and Visually Handicapped. I had a two-page list of novels I wanted. Some I'd read before and longed to be back in, and other, newer books, I'd jealously watched others reading around me. "Yep, we have that one," he said with a cheery cadence each time I gave him a title. I wanted to stay on the phone with Dennis forever. I wanted to tell him he was making all the difference.

"How many can I have at once?" I asked.

"There's no limit."

Everything else had a limit: the number of times a day I could navigate the stairs at home (two), the number of chores I could do in a row (one). Hope swelled so big in my chest I could barely talk. I would get through this. I would read, disappear, follow the lives of others who struggled and persevered. I would be lifted out of this broken body and deposited into one that worked for hours at a time. This would save me.

Dennis mailed me a ten-pound audio cassette player and every book on tape I'd asked for. I slid the four track tape into the faded yellow machine covered in braille bumps and curled up around it on the bed and pushed the extra large play button.

The voice swirled around me, hard to catch. Sentences broke in two. The story wouldn't put itself together in my mind. I kept hitting the huge rewind button to catch what I had missed, my head throbbing with the concentration required. I hit stop, shoved the cassette player, all the tapes, and that hateful hope balloon under the bed.

■ ■ ■

Six months after my dad died, the dreams started.

He walked into my freshman dorm room and found the vodka I'd hidden in the closet. "Obvious hiding place," he said with a look that said: Can't you do better than that?

"You're dead," I pointed out. "You can see through walls."

He laughed at the idea of it. "I'm not dead, I've just been busy." He shifted his feet, same worn jeans and old T-shirt. He lit a cigarette, squinted at me through the smoke. "Vodka is dumb. Drink whiskey."

A few months later, he was walking the beach in Maine in my dream, explaining patiently that he wasn't dead, he just wanted to live at the beach. Alone.

My brother had the same dreams. Dad would show up, and my brother would demand to know where he'd been all this time. Dad wouldn't say much but each time made it clear that he wasn't dead, that he'd just been out doing stuff. Like marrying other people and having other children. Or he'd just been out fly fishing. For a really long time.

This went on for a decade for both my brother and me. We got used to it.

One day, my brother sent me an email with the subject line: Found him!

Inside was a link to a *National Geographic* story about a home-steading family in the South Pacific. The dad of the family stared out at me from the photo of the family on the beach with a heart stopping resemblance—he was the right age, the right build, had the right spark in his eye. There he was, doing something that fit him much better than our house in a neighborhood ever had. And he looked happy. Like he used to on those firelit story nights.

In that first year in Alaska, I found him. Not in my dreams or on the pages of a magazine. In real life. On a four-wheeler.

My friend owned a falling down shack on a peninsula outside Glacier Bay, where a small group of homesteaders were living. Naturally, I wanted to go see it. We landed on a dirt runway after the Cessna pilot did a low sweep to scare off any animals large enough to crash into. As we strapped on backpacks and the plane roared off behind us back to town, the Alaskan version of my father pulled up, pistol strapped to his hip.

"Hey, Adam," he called out to my friend as he cut the engine.

The edges of the world went hazy, and my heart pounded in my throat as I took in the wide face, the playful eyes I'd missed with a fierceness big enough to swallow me up.

A grin spread across Adam's face. "You fishing?" He nodded at the gun at my Alaskan father's hip. It's not legal to shoot salmon, but it's a whole lot faster.

"Nah," the man said, his face breaking into the wide smile that had lit up my childhood. The skin across his cheekbones was smooth and red-tan, the wrinkles at his eyes and mouth were deep and well worn. And his eyes. They froze up my lungs. They were the same icy blue. He leaned across the four-wheeler and held out a hand to me. "Kenny."

I took the wide leathered hand I'd held a thousand times before. I wanted the time warp to stop, and I wanted it to go on forever.

The raw need for whoever has been ripped out of your life cannot be Processed or Talked Through or Worked On. The best you can do is let the years bury it so that you can accomplish the ordinary things in life, build an ordinary existence.

But when the extraordinary reaches out its hand, you take it. You look directly at what you have avoided, into the eyes of all you have lost. You accept the way the loss still cuts you in half, and probably always will, and realize all the things you've somehow managed to do anyway. You nod back when he smiles and says, "Good to see you," even though he has never seen this grown up version of you, or maybe has seen you all along.

■ ■ ■

Forty hours a week, I wrote down temperatures in the lab and rewrote the fishing book. For months, I hid from the world in this way. When I got to the end of the handwriting, I printed out the pages Mike had typed up and read one paragraph at a time. I held the words in my head, paced the dusty concrete floors with my noise canceling headphones on, and repeated sentence after sentence, memorizing the changes that made the sentences arc and flow, or made what I was trying to say more exact. I repeated the changes in my head and then went back to the printed page, making the changes as fast as possible. There was only so much looking at a page the dizziness allowed, and I had a lot of hours to fill in which I wanted to be on that pretend boat and not on land that moved like a boat.

Each day, I'd hand over pages of typed up manuscript with scribbled changes for Mike to incorporate into the Word doc. We worked our way through to the end of a full revision. We finished the same week I officially withdrew from school.

I didn't own a printer, so I waited until I got to work, then I waited until 10:00 p.m., when no one else was around, opened up the email on my work computer, and hit print. I wanted to walk around and hold it. A whole book I had written, a whole world imagined with a beginning, middle, and end. I'd sat in the white chairs on the deck in my cabin in Alaska with the first draft pressed to my chest in just such a way after hiking in gas to run the generator to run the printer in the cabin. But this was different. This was monumental. This was me swerving back out into the proper lanes of the highway despite the broken-down bike and no legs.

The printer on the test center floor remained slumped and quiet while I stared at it. I must've accidently sent it to another printer. I checked the next closest printer in the supply chain. Nothing.

An illegally printed, 350-page book with my name at the top of every page wasn't going to make me anyone's favorite night shift girl. The fear of losing my job when insurance was a mere eight weeks away pounded through me. I sprinted from floor to floor, from big printer to big printer, and then I started sneaking around the private offices until I found all 350 pages of my book in the CFO's office. I snatched it off his printer, sprinted out of carpet land back down to the echoey lab. I hugged the pages to my chest and spent the last hour of my shift with the stupidest of all stupid grins on my face.

I had heard that it often took sending a book to seventy-five agents to find one who wanted it so I (handwrote) a query letter that Mike typed up and, in my allotted ten-minute windows of computer time, queried seventy-five agents over the next many, many night shifts.

■ ■ ■

In the harsh hours I spent outside the world of my book, I thought vaguely through the foggy haze that a different, more intense structural approach might work. The only thing I knew about Rolfing was that it left bruises. It made sense somehow that chasing the dizziness out would require bruising.

I followed the address the nearest Rolfer gave me and found her in a cramped upstairs apartment. The couch and TV had been shoved up against the wall, and a massage table stood in the middle of the stuffy, knickknack filled living room. When she told me she was from a fishing family on the Kenai Peninsula, I felt perhaps it was destiny.

She patted the massage table with the wide, thick hands of fishermen. I lay down, my face in the hole. My forehead began to sweat as I watched the brown, nubbly carpet slosh underneath like the sea.

There was something of Alaska in her aggression. As she pushed, everything hurt and spun, and whatever last tether I had to my physical body slipped its mooring. I floated away. The only reprieve.

I didn't stick around to watch my battered body get battered some more. I traveled as far away as I could until she called me back and it started to get weird that I wasn't moving yet.

As I eased onto my feet, all the muscle that she had separated and moved lit up. I wrote out a check for her, my hand shaking. If it had been five dollars more, it would've bounced.

Some sessions, the Alaskan Rolfer was able to calm the dizziness, and at others, she stirred it up so bad I had to curl tight in the back seat of my car for indeterminate amounts of time before I could drive home. I wanted to stop seeing her, I needed to stop writing her checks, but every time another appointment rolled around, I got hooked by that one sliver of possibility that she would ease the dizziness, that this one time she might even cure it. Alaska is full of unexplainable powerful things.

■ ■ ■

I got so thin that a seven-year-old told me I looked gross.

Women said things like, "I wish I'd get dizzy to drop some of this weight."

I stopped wearing my seat belt.

I turned into that X-ray, flesh faded out, butterfly bones blurring into obscurity.

■ ■ ■

The acupuncturist filled an entire yellow legal pad with hand scribbled notes about me and moved on to a second legal pad. She cared. I could see it in the tilt of her head, the gentle hand on my knee. She hated the way the dizziness stayed just out of her reach. She mixed up herbs, offered me a reduced rate for appointments, clucked over the bruising from the Rolfer, and suggested her own chiropractor.

Her chiropractor was a lanky man who looked like he needed a steak. One of those ultramarathon runners that looks a little sick.

At the first appointment, it took so long to explain the whole story that we ran out of time for the manipulation. He held up a long thin finger. "I'll be right back," he said. "Other patients," he mumbled.

As the door clicked shut, I stared out at the expansive view of the mountains through the large windows of the exam room. The sun was setting, and the roads were full of people rushing on with their lives, most of them cocooned in good health. *I need to make a spreadsheet*, I thought. Something to hand over to save myself the exhaustion of explaining it. The reds turned to blues in the sky outside. I closed my eyes and fell instantly asleep in the quiet room.

Eventually, the acupuncturist's chiropractor came back. I wasn't sure how much time had passed. It was dark now. He bustled in, immediately wrapped his hands to my head, and located the pressure between C1 and the occipital. I didn't want him to slam the bones back into place. I was disoriented from sleeping. Everything was so fragile, and I was so tired. *I need to leave*, I thought. *Stand up*, I told myself as he wiggled my head to loosen it before the violence of the correction. Instead, I followed the protocol. I closed my eyes and let a random man do things to my body I didn't want done.

■ ■ ■

Late at night, in the dark.

ME: "It's like you're dating an old person."

MIKE: "I'm older than you."

ME: "I don't get why you stick around."

MIKE: "You're the most interesting person I've ever met."

ME: "This isn't interesting."

MIKE: "Right. This isn't. You are."

ME: "You should leave. Save yourself."

MIKE: "That'd be lame."

There's a picture from my twenty-fifth birthday party of Mike and me. We were just friends back then. My three-year-old cousin had been given a Polaroid camera, and she took her job as event photographer very seriously. My eight-year-old cousin had appointed himself bartender for the evening and made sure everyone milling around the backyard had a brand new ice cold beer in one hand before they finished the one in their other hand. An entire summer evening documented from a three-year old's height, everyone double fisting, Mike and I loose and happy, the world not spinning around us.

I dug the picture out, tucked it into the mirror above the dresser but then had to put it away. There was so much promise in the slanted, sepia toned, fun evening. The past calling out what could've been, shining a bright light on all that the future turned out not to be.

■ ■ ■

On the day my insurance started working, I went to a bar in the middle of the day and ordered a whiskey. It was worth the five minutes of liquid release before the dizziness came crashing back in, angry as a rattlesnake.

The second day I had insurance, I drove to a trailhead, managed to walk about a hundred yards, and sat on a rock in the sunshine. The wind bent the tall grass, and the sky stretched out forever. I took stock. I felt like a person who had just won the lottery, figuring out how I was going to spend the first million.

CHAPTER SEVEN

"How'd it go with my chiropractor?" the acupuncturist asked. I saw her two days a week for the dizzy drain. And for company.

I pressed my lips together and shook my head infinitesimally. Her face creased. "Maybe something gentler? How about cranial sacral therapy?"

I'd never heard of cranial sacral therapy, had no idea the bones of the head could be manipulated, but I found a PT who specialized in it and who took insurance.

She kept the lights low, and her hands were so gentle I began to trust her almost as much as I trusted the acupuncturist. She told me about her kids, her life outside work in a way that didn't require much from me. I slid into her life twice a week, pretended that one day I too would have a nice husband and a couple kids and healthy dinners in the freezer I spent all day Sunday preparing for the week because life was too busy—with important work helping people, kids sports after school, and fun evenings out with friends—to cook during the week.

Her hands spread across my skull, locating some sort of pressure valve, stilling the room, calming the way my head pounded, opening up room to think. Until the minute she removed her hands and everything sealed up tight again.

■ ■ ■

My mistake on climbing into the Cessna with Noel on that brisk summer morning in Alaska way before the dizziness showed up was in saying, "Don't spill the milk. It's open."

Noel was one of two pilots contracted to fly the Forest Service field crews out of our small town into the expansive national forest that surrounded it. Noel had flown in Vietnam and liked to listen to one song per flight, piped through everyone's headsets at an excessive volume, on repeat. The other pilot was known to be a bit safer, so crews that planned ahead typically locked in flights with him. My field partner, Natalie, and I had been flying with Noel most of the summer.

After a season on the tourist boat, I'd found a job on a wildlife crew trying to document stands northern goshawks were nesting in so that the timber crews would leave a few measly trees standing around the nest in a half-assed effort to protect the species.

Noel was lanky, Native Alaskan, and he owned a tanning bed. He was flying us out to a barge we used as a field camp that was currently anchored up on the north side of an island slated for timber sale. We would spend the next week hiking endless transects across the deeply forested, mountainous island, playing a recording of a territorial goshawk through a loudspeaker normal people bring to college football games, with the hope that a goshawk already on a nest would attack us. Then, we would tear through the forest, trying to tail him back to his nest, GPS his tree, and tell the timber guys to make other plans.

I said the thing about the milk as I was buckling into the passenger seat. Noel was easing us out of his hanger at the docks. We all pulled on headsets when he started up the deafening engine. He pushed levers in, pulled others out, turned some dials, and then turned them back. There were no screens on his control panel, just knobs and toggles. Our shoulders were one inch apart. Just before he pulled out into the channel with all the boats he'd have to take off around, he looked over and grinned, "You said the milk carton is open?"

All the food we'd need for the week was in cardboard boxes six feet behind us in the back of the plane. "Yeah," I said. "Well, sort of closed. It's one of those—" I mimicked opening one of those old school milk cartons from elementary school. The kind you pull half the top ridge apart and pop out the V to pour.

"Ahh . . ." he nodded, understanding. He looked around for commercial fishing boats coming and going between the harbor and the narrow channel that ran along the west side of the island we all lived on.

"Why'd you open it before packing it?" he asked.

"I needed milk for my coffee this morning and I was all out." I felt more than saw Natalie roll her eyes from the back seat. I always needed milk for my coffee, and a proper pillow on camping trips.

The narrow, rocky channel was marked by green and red buoys. It was summer, so the fishing fleet was back and forth from the fishing grounds to town to sell fish, refuel, and restock. To buy everyone a round at the bar or hang out, hoping someone else would. Noel peered into the hazy rain as we rocked in the short chop of the channel. He squinted out his side window, checked a dial or two, and decided which way was better to take off. He had two good choices.

The channel was barely a quarter mile across on a high tide and half that on a low. I only half trusted that Noel wouldn't try it anyway. I readjusted in the soft seat, pulled my knees back so they didn't accidentally hit any of the toggles on my side. The plane was rigged so that a copilot could take over if the pilot passed out or died, but I wasn't a copilot and neither was Natalie. It was all up to Noel.

My heart sped up a bit as Noel pointed us to the north. I liked the taking off part. The way town would fall away below us, nothing but mountains and valleys and ocean opening up in front of us. What I didn't like was when we inevitably flew through low hanging patches of fog and clouds. Noel always said he knew right where all the mountains were, but he said a lot of things.

He reached across me to the CD player Velcroed to the narrow rim between the front window and the passenger side door. He hit play, and Shania Twain filled up my head. Noel eyed the fifty-foot troller barreling straight for us in the channel. He hit the throttle, and everything began to shake as the pontoons pounded into the waves. The shake turned into a high pitched whine as we got on step, the huge steel bow of the boat getting bigger and bigger.

Noel was leaned forward in his seat. "C'mon, c'mon," he coaxed the plane that was twice my age.

My breath stalled out as we skipped across the tops of the waves. Shania hit a clear high note as Noel lifted us over the bow, a bearded raincoated man on deck, both arms in the air, yelling up at us. And then the smooth arc of swinging around the nearest mountain, following a dark green valley split in half by a river I loved to fish.

Noel reached over and set the round CD player to repeat. Since the music was too loud to talk over, I watched the landscape crinkle and flow beneath me. There was a power to it. To every day spent in it. A place where, of course, everything could go wrong in one second. A place where people carried that knowledge with them in the hang of their wet clothes. A place where it hovered in the background of conversations. A place where no one pretended otherwise.

After an exceptionally smooth flight, the barge came into view. But Noel didn't initiate the descent that would set us down on the water next to it. Instead, he flew over the top of the barge, straight for the wall face of the mountain at the terminus of the bay.

"Noel!" I said, reaching out to push all the buttons on the CD player, meaning to turn it off so he could hear me.

He banked hard right, which caused my hands to fly back to the seat, the only thing to hang on to. His lips moved along with Shania as he banked even more until I was looking straight down at the ocean through my side window. There was nothing but sky out his window, and at the edge of mine, the rock wall, way too close. We did some sort of roll that rocketed all my organs up against my spine and then settled on the water next to the barge, facing the way we'd come.

Noel reached across and hit stop, whipped off his headset, and jumped out of the plane as we bumped up against the dock while I was breathing in my nose and out my mouth, swallowing all the extra spit my body was suddenly making.

Noel whipped a fancy knot around the cleat, tying the plane to the barge.

By the time I crawled over his seat and out of the plane, he had both our backpacks and both boxes of food on the dock. He winked as he untied the plane and pushed off the dock with one foot, "Go on, then. Check it."

I peeked in the food box. Everything around the milk was splashed with it.

"It spilled."

He had one hand on the door, one foot in. He grinned. "Of course it did! We went upside down!" He cracked himself up.

The water lapped at the edge of the barge. The hollow silence of the woods pressed in around us before Noel cut it in half with the sharp kick of his engine starting.

I stood on the dock and stared after him. I'd spent the years of college with a red Solo cup in my hand, feeling like Shrek in a land full of humans. I nodded and listened as they talked about how the new boyfriend was definitely the one, about the job their dad's partner had offered them right out of college that would lead to all the necessary promotions, about the top of the line mountain bike they were going to get next. Noel made so much more sense to me than any of them ever had. If you deeply accept that life can go sideways at any given time and you invest in your ability to manage when it does instead of investing in controlling that it never goes sideways, there's less fear and more room to actually live. If you can die in the dirt of a ball field at forty-five, then why not flip a Cessna upside down to spill milk just because you can?

■ ■ ■

The ophthalmologist kept her hands buried in the deep rectangular pockets of her buttoned up, white doctor coat. It was dim in the exam room, which always helped, but the chair was reclined too far. I wanted to stand, shake her hand, meet her eye to eye. Instead, I slumped in the way the chair demanded with my belly exposed.

"What can I help you with?" She towered over me, even though she was shorter than me.

"I've been dizzy for a year and a half." I handed her the multipage spreadsheet.

"And you came to an ophthalmologist?" She looked at me like I'd handed her a mayonnaise sandwich.

"My eyes jump. All the time. I just thought . . . well . . ." I saw myself through her eyes: Stupid. Begging for help. Submissive. "It's all there. In the spreadsheet." I willed myself not to run out of the room.

She read through the spreadsheet slowly. Her forehead creased as she vacuumed up every word, and I thought, *Oh, thank god, a scientific brain at work. She will find the regularity in the irregular pattern.* Coming here hadn't been stupid, it had been creative.

She set the spreadsheet down on the small desk with the computer. I looked at her expectantly. From deep in her pockets, she pulled out the heavy handled, super bright flashlight thing all eye doctors love. She peered long and slow and deep into one eye and then into the other.

She twisted away from me and flipped the overhead light on in one quick motion that left me blinking and the room sloshing.

"There is nothing wrong with your eyes," she said with a one shouldered shrug. "Perfectly normal," she said as she picked up my spreadsheet and thrust it in my direction. "You cannot fix a problem at C1."

If you are typically moved to tears when someone tells you a sad story, people generally aren't like, *Hey, you should probably go to medical school*. You are encouraged to consider medicine if you get top scores in math and science, if you are good at memorizing facts. There is a certain security in the idea that if X, then Y holds true. But the whole of medicine is like the whole of life. There are times when you spray a bear in the face with pepper spray and he goes away, and there are other times when you spray a bear in the face with pepper spray and he attacks. If X, then Y is false security. There is chaos in life, and there is chaos in the human body. We can memorize and plan all we want, but there are always times when we are forced to improvise.

I wanted to say all this, but it rubbed up against all those boundaries. If she'd never been trapped in everyday dizziness, how could she ever see the necessity of working outside what she'd always done? If she wasn't willing to feel the desperation that necessitated the stretch, how was she ever going to be willing to stretch into thinking differently? If she was safe in healthy land, why would she ever cross over into sick land to see it my way? Better to just make sick land go away.

I took the spreadsheet, balanced for a minute with my feet on the floor before I let go of the chair, and ran a hand along the wall to stay upright on my way out.

■ ■ ■

I had a stalker once. In college. He had a class across the hall from me that got out at the same time. He would wait, leaned up against the wall, and follow me out. He was thin, quiet, and moody. Oversized, overworn T-shirt and heavy boots. Never too close, but always there. He slowly figured out the rest of my class schedule and would be waiting outside those classrooms too to trail me for a while.

He showed up at my house once. Walked a slow circle around it while I bolted around inside, locking all the windows and doors. He left careful footprints in the snow that taunted me for days.

The ophthalmologist's words stalked me in the same way, always waiting for me in the in-between places, following silent and sulky somewhere behind me. The threat of them always with me. If there was no way to solve a problem at C1 and that was the only problem ever identified by more than one doctor, then I was condemned.

I changed my patterns, slipped through new doorways trying to ditch the ophthalmologist's words, strung out even more by the added vigilance.

The cranial-sacral therapist moved slower, as if she somehow could sense this new instability. Barely moving, her hands relieved the pressure between the bones of my skull, between the frayed and frantic parts of my mind. I showed up twice a week for months, the copay pennies, in desperate need of the relief that she could provide for a few short minutes. Each time, within minutes of her letting go, the dizziness rushed back in. By the time I was in the parking lot, the dizziness was typically throwing punches, angered by the way she'd tied its hands with hers.

We never talked about it, but she and I both knew she was holding me a few steps back from the ledge. I crouched there. Rested.

■ ■ ■

Of the seventy-five agents I queried, fifteen asked to read the whole fishing book. This was back in the day of sending actual pages in the mail. I made sure my work computer was connected to the big printer in the test center, waited until everyone else had gone home, and printed. The weight of the novel in my hands pierced through the fog of dizziness with something akin to happiness.

"Another rejection," I said to Mike one afternoon. I was sitting at the dining room table, checking my email. I swallowed against the disappointment and read the email:

Dear Rachel,

You've got a great eye for detail and setting, great character dynamics and development but the voice just didn't sit well with me. I'm going to have to pass on this one.

"I never liked her anyway," Mike said from the couch.

"You don't even know who that's from." My email dinged. "Oh! Here's another reply." My heart soared with the possibility that this could be it. I opened the next email and read it out loud:

Dear Rachel,

Great prose, but I wasn't swept up in the plot and Ellie didn't develop quite the depth I'd hoped.

"She chews with her mouth open. You don't want her for an agent anyway," Mike said, making me laugh despite the sting of having hoped. I wondered if it was better to not hope at all. I also wondered what kind of sadist I might be to be throwing myself into a second underworld full of people turning cold shoulders in the face of my clear, apparent, desperate desire.

■ ■ ■

Four days later, my phone rang, which is how I learned that if an agent really wants your book, they call rather than email. I signed on the dotted line with an aggressive grandma of an agent.

"What revisions are you thinking?" I asked in a follow-up phone call a few days later. I'd heard agents typically want a lot of revisions, which would take me forever in my one paragraph at a time process, but whatever, I would just lean into the dizziness harder with whatever I had left.

"No revisions," she said. "Let's just sell it."

Grandmas always just know.

She wrote me update emails in all lower case, no punctuation, like ee cummings.

sent to ten editors yesterday, twelve more this morning

A future crystallized despite all the fog. There would be a book in the world with my name on it. I would Achieve Anyway.

■ ■ ■

The only appointment I could get at the ultra-expensive-unless-you-have-insurance Spine Center was during rush hour. Mike was at work, and the one-eyed driving business was seeming less like perseverance and more like stupidity, so I asked my friend Erin to take me down to Denver.

Hope glinted in the sun like fool's gold as I imagined the top-notch medical care I was about to receive. I could see the specialist in my mind's eye. His efficiency. His gleaming office. His Ivy League educated mind focused on X-rays he'd be able to take in his office and read immediately. No lowbrow, *Head on over to the hospital, we'll call you later* kind of X-raying situation.

I was right about the gleaming waiting room. A whole Costco box of Pledge, monthly, no question.

"Want me to come in with you?" Erin asked.

"Sure."

The semester we spent aboard the sailboat, Erin and I used to climb up the rigging and sit on the topsail beam a hundred feet in the air in twenty-foot seas. We used to plot the course of the ship using a sextant and the sun and the stars. We used to steer through thirty-foot waves in the black of night.

We sat down in the over-air-conditioned waiting room in two cloth chairs.

"This sucks," she said after forty-five minutes of waiting.

"Yeah," I said, although I'd hardly noticed. My internal frustration meter had adjusted over the years to not switch on until somewhere around the hour mark of waiting on doctors.

We were called back to an exam room, and the doctor bustled in, eventually. Something about the belt and shoes suggested his country club membership. His eyes never really landed on me. They skipped around—the computer, my face, Erin, the spreadsheet, back to the computer—as I answered his questions. I forced my way through the brain fog, the nausea. Erin watched me closer than normal. I'd talked to her some about the dizziness but not much. I rarely had the energy to hang out, much less invite someone else in to see the raw wound my life had turned into.

The afternoon a wind spout threatened to rip our sails to shreds four hundred miles from land, Erin and I had been the first to volunteer to climb over the bow of the boat, out onto the bowsprit, to lower the sails. The bowsprit punched through wave after wave as we lashed the jib topsail our crewmates were working the lines to drop. We stood on a loose wire over a raging sea, our chest harnesses keeping us tethered to the boat as we were plunged waist deep into each oncoming wave. The possibilities in our nineteen-year-old lives that day as endless and big as the sea surrounding us.

The doctor interrupted before I was done explaining the chiropractors, the C1 business, all the ENTs. "Can you describe the dizziness?"

"It's like seasickness, all the time. Walls like waterfalls. Floors sloshing around."

He pressed his lips together, ran his eyes over me, looking for his own evidence, it seemed. "It's bad," I added. I wanted to tell him about the snow covered fawn, how I still couldn't get it out of my mind. The pull of it as an answer getting stronger and stronger. Instead, I said, "I had to lay down on the floor of Costco."

He breathed out noisily. "Let's get an X-ray."

Sure enough, the X-ray room was across the hall. I put on the lead vest, held my breath as instructed while the tech ducked behind the wall out of danger's reach.

The doctor's medical assistant ushered me back into the exam room after the X-ray. She wore cartoon characters and soft shoes. "He'll be back in shortly," she said as she pulled the door closed. Erin had clearly been sitting there the whole time, boiling over. "It's like he didn't believe you," she said.

"I don't look sick."

"You don't look right." She got a look on her face like you do when someone says, *Smell this meat, do you think it's bad?* "But he doesn't know you," she went on. "You should quit with the poker face thing you always do and cry or something."

We both laughed at that. I am whatever the opposite of a crier is.

"I'm serious," she said. "You need to act the part."

I'd thought of this a number of times. Had considered the fact that perhaps I was a bad patient, a poor communicator, too stoic, too good at appearing put together. Perhaps if I indulged the horrible state I was in, let it leak out everywhere, I would be taken more seriously. Perhaps if I reinforced the expected power dynamics, everything would go more smoothly. Patient as out of control and dependent, doctor as in control and hero. But letting the dam break felt incredibly dangerous. I was just barely keeping it together enough to accomplish minimal tasks in life, if I let the dam break, I was certain I'd never survive. Which is what made me think perhaps they were all right, perhaps I needed more therapy. But in my dramatically reduced state, this was the way I was managing, and I did not have the energy to figure out any other way.

Twenty-five minutes later, the doctor came back with the X-ray, which he clicked into the backlit thing on the wall meant for this purpose. I averted my eyes from the image of myself fading away.

"Perfectly sound spine, as far as this X-ray shows. No problem at C1."

I missed whatever he said next. Had all those chiropractors been wrong? Were chiropractors and spine doctors always going to disagree? Was this guy wrong? Did anyone know what they were talking about?

"Mandy will take you back there," he said as he stood and stepped through the door just as the cartoon medical assistant stepped through it. A perfectly timed patient herding team.

"Where are we going?" I asked her.

"To schedule your MRI," she said, looking at the clipboard the doctor put in her hands as he passed her on his way to the next patient.

"I already had one. I can probably get the results sent over." She smiled kindly. "He likes to do his in house."

I relished the fact that because I now had insurance, I could follow her into a small office where a woman scheduled me for three weeks out. So easy.

■ ■ ■

Five weeks later, the MRI results were in. Mike was at work again and so was Erin, so I drove one-eyed in the middle of the day. The spine doctor bustled into the exam room, starched plaid shirt tucked in tight. "How are you?" he asked with a glance as he sat down, rolled up to the computer screen, and reached for the mouse.

"Okay," he barreled on, apparently oblivious or perhaps just expecting that I would remain silent in the face of this ridiculous question. "Just pulling up your test results." My palms started to sweat. I tried to brace myself for the inevitable *There's nothing to be done*. For the coming shrug.

The computer screen flickered, and he began to scroll and click at breakneck speed. I looked away to keep from puking. I stared at his hairline instead. It was perfectly even and trim at his neckline, like the horizon at sea but not nearly as calming.

He breathed out a forced breath, abandoned the mouse, and turned to face me. He looked at me for the first time, smiled, and folded his hands in his lap. "All normal," he said, his face lit up like high noon in the desert. I wanted to scream at him that this was clearly nothing to smile about. I sat in the hard plastic chair and tried to get my mind to line up some sort of response. There was nothing normal about the situation at all.

Why was it so hard to communicate in the clinical setting? I have no idea. Something to do with the brain fog, my constitution, with the energy it takes to cross men in power, with the way the world and all the healthy people in it had stretched out of my reach.

There are bays in southeast Alaska with a specific kind of sucking mud. There are big tides, plenty of chances where you beach your skiff on a low tide with a huge stretch of mud between you and the line of trees on solid shore. Cautionary tales abound about people who think, *It's just mud. I can walk across it.* Which is true, most of the time, but if you happen to be in one of those certain bays with that certain mud, you will not be able to walk across it. You will sink in above the boots, above the knees, above the waist, and the mud will compress such that you cannot lift your legs out of it. There are stories of men stuck up to their waists, drowned as the tide comes back in, and one particularly horrible legend about a helicopter brought in to try to pull someone out, to horrific results.

With the spine doctor and so many other doctors, I felt like I was constantly saying, *Look, it's not that kind of mud, it's this kind of mud. And no, I cannot just pull my feet out like you can in most mud.* I felt like I was frantically pointing at the changing tide, the way it was gathering itself out in the channel, beginning to move back in.

The cartoon lady opened the door and murmured something. The spine doctor stood up. "Excuse me," he said and followed her out into the hallway.

The door clicked, and my vision blacked at the edges. Because I didn't know what else to do, and because my limbs had turned to wet sand, I continued to sit there.

The cartoon popped back through the door, ponytail flying. "Okay, the doctor wants to schedule a cortisone shot next. Let's go ahead and find a day and time that works. You'll have to go to the hospital for that," she said brightly, turning to the computer.

"But why . . ." I could only get the first two words to line up.

"Not the most comfortable procedure," she bubbled on. "A shot in your spine. But you'll be fine to drive yourself home afterward."

I was anything but fine to drive myself anywhere.

"He said everything looked normal. Why would I need a cortisone shot?"

She hunched over a multicolored scheduler on the screen. "That's his treatment plan. Thursday the twenty-eighth at noon work for the shot?"

I wanted to fight back, to understand, to reason. A needle in my spine seemed so drastic. But there was that pathetic sliver of hope. "Can I talk to him again?"

"He's in with another patient." Her straight hair glinted like metal in sunlight.

"I'll wait."

She pressed her lips together until they turned white. "I'm afraid he's all booked up the rest of the day. Thursday the twenty-eighth at noon work for the cortisone shot?"

I nodded, and she all but bubble lettered the day and time onto a card and handed it to me before ushering me out of the office.

■ ■ ■

What I had to do: spend fifteen minutes online signing up for the spine doctor's patient portal in order to compose a short message (only one hundred characters allowed) to ask him why in god's name I needed a cortisone shot in my spine. Wasn't it super dangerous to stick a needle in a spine? Wasn't there a risk of paralysis? It all seemed utterly not necessary. Except that maybe he suspected, but ran out of time to tell me, some other diagnosis that would not show up on an MRI or X-ray but would be cured by cortisone.

What signing up for the patient portal and composing a hundred-character-long question cost me: hours in which the room kaleidoscoped, the bed rolling under me and the window stretching away from me, Alice in Wonderland-like, until the outside world was miles away.

■ ■ ■

The spine doctor had still not written back two weeks later when it was time to get the cortisone shot. I called the office and was told the only way to discuss matters with him was to make another appointment for three weeks out or to contact him through the patient portal.

I paced just out of sight of the big desk at the hospital, where I was to check in for the cortisone shot, and tried to ignore the way that horrible hope illuminated the possibility that I would walk over to the desk, check in, get the shot, and walk out of there not dizzy.

Because I could not bear to think I might miss my opportunity to get out of jail due to fear, I took a deep breath and stepped into the airy, open waiting room with big, swoopy, decorative architecture above and below the front desk. Why couldn't architects just design things with straight fucking lines? The seasickness increased as I sailed out into the middle of the swoopy room.

I checked in and sat down in a row of chairs. The way to survive a body is to disassociate the mind. But it wasn't working. I could not stop thinking about a needle entering my spine. Shouldn't I have gotten a handout outlining the potential risks? What if they paralyzed me? They'd shrug and tell me to get a wheelchair. That's what.

Desperation was coming at me from all sides like a pit of snakes.

"Rachel Weaver," a woman in pale blue scrubs called from a door that led into the depths.

I stood. The snakes writhed.

I caught the eye of the woman in blue scrubs. She smiled. I turned away, found the exit of the hospital, and burst out into the parking lot, my chest heaving as if the charging bear had just veered off at the last minute.

■   ■   ■

The GP, who drove a Subaru, went by her first name, and brought her dog to work in the converted Victorian home, went through my spreadsheet line by line in the dim light of a lamp on her desk in what was once the back porch.

"I need help figuring out what type of doctor to see next." I studied her studying the typed up version of my misery, wondering if all she saw was provider, diagnosis, result or if she could sense the deer, sense the fact that I was wild with the knowledge that I would have to let Mike go, that I couldn't possibly subject him to a limited life, the clear ringing desperation over the fact that I would never again carry a heavy pack in a dense wood.

She took her readers off. "This is an exhaustive list."

The defeated cadence of the words crawled up my back like the soft legs of a spider.

I get that doctors need to put up walls for sanity. You can't go through your day crying with every patient. It's the boundaries that keep them safe, keep things ordered and the day moving along. Besides, what kind of idiot beaches their boat in the bay with the human swallowing mud and then expects someone to come out into it to save them?

She took a deep breath. "There's nothing else to do at this point." She dropped her readers on the desk, pinched at the top of her nose between her eyes. "You're just going to have to learn to live with it."

■ ■ ■

Later, at midnight, on my way home from work, the wooden arm at the train tracks stopped me on a two lane road next to a farm. There was no way I could live with it. It was asking too much. As the train pounded past, its power rattling up through my feet, I thought, *Here. Late at night. Like this. It would be over so fast.*

CHAPTER EIGHT

Still plagued by the fact that it made good sense that a neck stiff as concrete might cause dull headaches and dizziness, I found a chiropractor who specialized in upper cervical manipulation. He was younger than me, fresh faced, and a little nervous.

I followed him behind one of those Japanese room dividers in a single roomed, white walled office free of furniture and tried to convince myself that there was no problem with him being painfully young. He was fresh from school, his head filled with the latest research.

I sat on the ubiquitous brown table of healers while he rolled a handheld cold metal contraption down my spine. Through my shirt, thank goodness. He was too young to request one of those gowns that gaped open at the back. I wondered how accurate the instrument was through fabric. I tried not to feel sad for him and for me as we both submitted ourselves to questionable science in a hollow room. The handheld contraption was attached to the computer by a long cord and eventually displayed my spine, with big patches of red up near my neck.

"This here is your problem area," he said.

Obviously.

After the violence, we were back to the cold roller. "All green now," he said, all smiles and flushed cheeks.

I looked around. A person checking the damage after an accident. The room was a bit stiller, I could think a bit more clearly, my dull, all-the-time headache was vaguely better.

I forgave the chiropractor his youth and came back twice a week for months. I kept giving him my credit card. He bought potted plants, curtains, a surrealist painting. He made me worse as often as he made me better, but I was hooked like a junkie willing to lose everything in search of the high because every so often, he would shove me above the surface of the churning water and I would gasp, fill my lungs, and feel just enough hope to survive the next drag down into the depths.

■ ■ ■

The rejections peppered my inbox:

. . . delightful writing, good dialogue and description, great development of secondary characters, but I just didn't fall in love with it . . .

. . . strong voice, great storyline, but just doesn't match my list . . .

. . . exceptional in many ways. The voice is engaging, excellent writing, but overall I felt the novel could have accomplished more . . .

. . . great description of place but overall the story was too slow . . .

■   ■   ■

I pulled the chair over to the glass door that looked out at the parking lot at work and watched my favorite hawk. He was pissed as usual. When the HR lady left for the night, he screamed at her. When one of the engineers left, he false swooped him. *Right,* I thought, *right.* In the face of endless pavement, huge buildings, cars, people everywhere, he remained adamant that there was still a line that he would not allow crossed. What did it matter what anyone in pantyhose in New York thought of my book? That wasn't the point.

I waited until everyone left work, stole a stack of paper from the copier, and started a story about Jess and Marta, two outcasts with nothing but gumption who take down the whole of the Forest Service timber industry.

■   ■   ■

Healthy people my own age frolicked at the opposite end of a very long tunnel. I could see them, but it was too hard to yell through the tunnel, to connect in any other way except to watch them with longing. I began to understand old people. The way they were focused on the malfunctions of their body. Consumed by it. My heart ached in a new way when I saw a man in a wheelchair, a woman with a constant tremor, a guy begging for money with wild eyes. These were my people. The ones who lived beyond the edges of everyone else. The ones consumed with things much more unwieldy than the difficult boss, the upcoming bills, what to make for dinner, how bad the ski traffic would be that weekend.

A hot hatred began to boil. For anyone I saw reading a book as if it were no big deal. For a coworker who went on and on about a new boyfriend who maybe wasn't as into it as she was. For my neighbor who complained he'd been sick with the flu for *an entire week*. I wanted to punch them all in the throat. I wanted to zap them into my existence for one hour and watch them freak out.

I became quick friends with a woman over seventy when she mentioned she struggled with "dizzy spells." We were sitting in the back seat of a mutual friend's car together when she first mentioned it.

"Me too," I whispered.

Her eyes flashed, and I felt she understood me in a way no one else ever had. "How often?" she asked.

"All the time."

She gasped. "Who do you see?"

"I can't find anyone to help."

She pulled out a small notebook, began scribbling, ripped out the page, and handed it to me.

"The Center for Dizziness," it read, with a street address that wasn't far away.

"Go there," she said.

"I've told twenty doctors I'm dizzy and not one has mentioned that there's something called the Center for Dizziness *within an hour's drive*?" I felt like I was going to choke.

She pursed her lips. "Doctors are like ants. They are all doing the same thing, but they don't talk to each other."

"I think ants talk to each other through pheromones."

She cocked her eyebrows. "Well, doctors don't have those."

I sank further back into the seat. "I wish they did."

She patted my knee. "Me too, dear."

■ ■ ■

Greenpeace had arrived in Alaska. And they were after us. We had to be prepared and on alert. The forest supervisor paced slowly at the front of the meeting room in her heavy heels and heavier green pants. In my time in small town Alaska, I'd learned that the Sierra Club and Greenpeace were not universally accepted as good. There were some others in that room who, like me, thought maybe the trees should be left standing, but they didn't speak up either.

I sat on my hard plastic chair with the rest of the seasonal field workers anxious to catch our flights or gas up the boat for a day hiking streams, tagging trees, or, in my case, looking for a goshawk that didn't want to be found.

The *Rainbow Warrior*, the forest supervisor went on to explain, was the Greenpeace battleship headed our way. They'd been shunned in ports to the south of us, refused fuel and water. Their response: Free beer to anyone who would come aboard.

Thirty minutes later, Natalie and I were loading up in the Cessna. Jake, the other pilot in town besides Noel, was thirtysomething and a fan of aviator glasses, even though it was cloudy three hundred days a year. He'd heard I was writing a novel based in southeast Alaska, which was true, and had decided it was a romance, which was not true.

Jake kept his plane in a hangar at the airport instead of in a hangar at the docks like Noel did. Which was a good decision on Noel's part. If he both took off and landed on the water, there was no messy business of having to remember if the wheels were up or down.

"Come clean," Jake was saying through the headset as I clipped the seat belt across my waist in the back seat. "Just tell me who the main character is based on. Jamie D, we cleared for takeoff?" He looked up the runway strip and down it. Scanned the skies above us.

Natalie, already in her seat belt and headset, sitting two inches to Jake's right, glanced back to see if I might spill the beans.

"Yeah, go ahead, Jake. Cleared for takeoff." It was too loud to talk while Jake rattled us down the runway and up into the air.

Once we were up and banking hard right to swing around in front of the fast approaching mountains, I said, "Love is a dead end road."

Jake was sitting right in front of me, his back pushing the front seat less than an inch from my knees. He looked over at Natalie and shook his head and dove us into a thick cloud bank. Before everything turned white, I took note of how we were over the middle of the channel, the mountains on either side a favorable distance away.

"You know, people like to read romance novels," Jake said. "You could probably make a lot more money if you just take whatever you've got and turn it into a romance. One starring a pilot." The inlets and bays below us snapped by in sharp flashes as we punched through billowing clouds.

"Finn McPherson thinks it should feature a lawn mower man." Finn ran the one landscaping business in town.

"The fuck?" Jake said. "A lawn mower man romance is going nowhere."

We burst through the clouds, and there it was. Anchored up in a secluded bay about twenty miles from town: the *Rainbow Warrior*.

All three of us sat up straight, straining to see as we flew right over the top of the dreaded pirate ship. It had a steel hull, clean lines, and a fresh coat of white paint. It sat big and powerful in the flat, gray water of the bay. Not a soul on deck.

Jake lifted us over a small hill and dropped toward the water in the neighboring bay that was slated for a timber sale. Natalie and I had been spending considerable time scouring the area. We'd found a goshawk that refused to lead us to his nest so we could protect it in the upcoming timber sale. As Jake lined up to touch down, he said, "I hear there's free beer on board."

"No one would know, way out here," Natalie said. She was born and raised in southeast Alaska but had lived in other parts of the world. I didn't know where Jake was from, only that he'd been in town a long time. It was impossible to guess how each of them felt about Greenpeace. I watched and waited. One thing I knew for sure: While politics were derisive on the small island, free beer was not.

"What time am I picking you two up?" Jake asked.

"4:30," I answered.

"Perfect." Jake cut the engine, and we glided on the small wake toward the soft shore. He hopped out his door, onto the float, pulled the oar from its latches, and steered until we were within a few feet of the beach. By the time I'd climbed over his seat and out his door, he had pulled our backpacks from the small hatch, and Natalie was wading to shore. He handed my pack over and smiled like the main character in a romance novel. "See you at happy hour."

I smiled at my reflection in his aviator glasses and stepped off the float into six inches of water. Not too high to top the boots. On the beach, Natalie and I strapped our packs on, watched Jake take off for town, and cut into the woods, staying on high olfactory alert for wet dog and/or patchouli.

At 4:15 p.m., we were back on the beach. We dropped our heavy packs, made heavier by how soaked through they both were. It had started raining midmorning and was still at it. We'd run into one bear, no goshawks, and no warriors. My thick rubber rain gear was wet from the inside out with sweat and from the outside in with rain from the wet, whipping branches of the blueberry shrub we'd spent much of the day bushwhacking through. My fingers were pruned like I'd been in the bathtub too long, and I was shivering hard enough that my shoulder blades seemed to be knocking together.

Natalie pulled out a *Vogue* magazine in a Ziplock bag and settled with her back against a big, dark rock.

"You brought the heaviest magazine you could find?"

"Shut up. *Vogue*'s awesome." She crossed her feet and settled the seven-pound magazine in her lap. "It just came in the mail this morning." She began to flip through the bright, glossy pages as if she were waiting for a flight in an airport.

I walked down the beach, lay down on the smooth, gray rocks, and rested in the big silence of the bay. My mind gave up its rusty circular patterns and stretched out over the smooth, gray water under the smooth, gray cloud ceiling. The sound of the water and the feel of the misty rain on my face untied the knots life in town had tied me in. I began to hope the beer was cold and had a blue ribbon on it.

"Hey!" Natalie looked up from a page in the magazine. "It says here you burn one hundred calories for every fifteen minutes you shiver!"

"Fantastic news," I called out. I ended up shivering at least half the days we worked in the field.

Jake's plane was the sound of a persistent mosquito at first. Ten minutes later, he touched down just offshore, jumped out onto the float, and used the oar to swing the plane sideways up to the beach. "They're gone!" he said as we waded out into the water.

I climbed into the plane behind Natalie and said, "Well, then, I hope you brought me a PBR."

"We'll take the long way home. Do some searching," Jake said as he settled into the pilot's seat.

We wound and banked and twisty turned until I started to think maybe a beer didn't sound too good after all.

"There!" Natalie pointed out her side window. I unbuckled and slid across the back seat to look out Natalie's side and spotted the white mammoth of a ship tied up at a timber loading dock at the terminus of a road that led to an active timber sale on an uninhabited island. Natalie and I had worked off that road most of the month of June, documenting goshawk nests. Jake dipped the wing so he could see too.

"That's not good," Jake said. He swooped us inland and dolphined over the top of the canopy, following the one and a half lane logging road. In the narrow strip the canopy allowed, several miles up, I spotted the lime green of two Forest Service vehicles parked haphazardly, a logging truck at a standstill, and several men yelling at each other.

Perched high above them on a three legged contraption that stretched across the entirety of the road, with a seat forty feet up, sat a warrior in a bike helmet. As we passed overhead, he looked up with that same beady eyed look goshawks get right before they aim their twenty-two-inch bodies straight for the head of anything they perceive as a threat.

"What the hell," I said as the whole scene whipped under us, and Jake pinned me to my seat as he pulled us straight up and over the tallest trees.

Jake glanced back over his shoulder at me. "They set those chair things up over the road so the log trucks can't get to the trees slated for extraction."

"Good way to get sent to the hospital," Natalie said through the headset as Jake banked hard left and then leveled us out, the ocean moving gray and cold underneath us. "Or the morgue."

Ballsy, I thought as I watched the landscape below map its way toward home. And here I am too chickenshit to say I love trees and I prefer them standing. I hated that goshawks got only a hundred-foot circle of protection when we found their nests, while the rest of the valley that held their food was clear-cut. But did I ever say anything? No. The pattern of me saying nothing lit up iridescent as I scrolled back through my life. My hands got fidgety. I wondered what it looked like perched up there, held aloft by nothing more than spindly poles and the thrill of wrestling power away from powerful forces with nothing more than your own ingenuity.

■ ■ ■

The Center for Dizziness was a collaboration between ENTs, vestibular PTs, and an ophthalmologist. Armed with my new insurance, I took the next available appointment. Three months later, I made the one-eyed drive to Denver.

The office was in a nondescript, four story brick building, at the end of a long hallway. Every few feet along the hallway hung computer generated artwork full of abstract, asymmetrical shapes. The kind of pictures you look at, if your eyes work correctly, and the image seems in motion. If you are dizzy, looking at this type of artwork makes you have to lie down on the floor. I kept my eyes focused straight ahead and wondered what kind of fucked up person picked out such artwork to hang along a hallway that leads to the Center for Dizziness.

I checked in, waited for twenty minutes, went through a hearing test, which I passed with flying colors, and then waited another forty minutes for the ENT who was to evaluate me first.

He was in his late fifties, had a belly, a thick, bushy mustache, and the wide, puffy face of alcoholics.

He sat on the rolly chair in front of me, and I thought, *Dad, if you are out there, please, please, please make this guy be the one who helps.*

The doctor smiled, which was nice, and said, "What can I do for you?"

"I've been dizzy every day for two years. I've seen a lot of doctors." I handed him my spreadsheet, which he glanced at for thirty seconds and set down. He settled his watery eyes back on me and waited. So I told him who I had seen and what they had each determined was not the problem. This took a while, which is why I made the spreadsheet. Somewhere in the midst of me explaining, his cell phone buzzed. He pulled it out of his pocket, read a text, and began texting back. I stopped talking and waited, thinking perhaps it was an emergency. Perhaps someone was in cardiac arrest in one of the other rooms.

"Keep talking," he said, eyes still on the screen, fingers tapping out a response. "It's just my wife."

Eventually, he put his phone away, let me spool out the rest of my energy finishing the long, drawn out story that was clearly written on the spreadsheet. When I finished, he looked in my ears. I wanted to skip this stupid step. I took Anatomy and Physiology. A vestibular issue lies locked away in the inner ear. But that was the ritual. As much a part of the visit as the forms with the swimming lines, the *Golf* and *People* magazines, the plug in waterfalls, the shrugs, the annoyance, the hurrying.

"Your hearing test came back normal, which suggests it's not Ménière's. There are two vestibular tests I'd like to run."

Good, I thought, *more data*. I forgave him the texting.

He pushed a red button on the wall I had not noticed, and a rail thin technician appeared within seconds, opening the door, ushering me out.

I checked my watch. The doctor and I spent seven minutes together, two of which he was on his phone.

The technician led me to another small room where he explained that he was going to alternately shoot air and then water into my ears while I wore thick, black goggles that would read my eye movements. "It's going to make you dizzy," he warned as he handed me the goggles to put on.

"I'm already dizzy," I said, fear creeping in at the corners.

He gave me a sad look. "Lay back."

The paper crinkled and stuck to my neck.

"Take this in case you feel sick." He picked up my hand and moved it to the metal edge of a bedpan sort of thing he'd balanced on my jutting hip bones. I couldn't see a thing. The goggles blacked out my vision.

"Ready?" he asked.

And then the impending test became the seven-hundred-pound brown bear stepping out of the blueberry shrub in front of me. There was the immediate understanding that I wouldn't come out on top, the flood of adrenaline, everything leaving my mind, all muscles screaming to *get away*.

I tore at the goggles and sat up, breathing hard. The tech was right next to me, tapping at the computer the goggles were attached to by a long cord. "Need a minute?" he asked, cocking his head but otherwise remaining slouched in the chair.

I gripped the metal bedpan thing, thinking I might throw up before it even began. But, I argued with myself, this test would tell me definitively if my inner ear was working correctly. They would find something, and this would be the end of all of it. I just had to suffer this, and then we'd know.

I lay back down and slowly replaced the goggles. Everything went black. Before the technician did anything, I was already spinning in outer space, alone. A hot, silent tear streaked down my cheek and into my ear.

"Alright, here goes." His voice was soft and close as he maneuvered something into my ear. I wanted him to hold my hand, assure me I would survive this, that the train tracks were a bad idea. But words like this always stuck in my throat. My abhorrence for appearing vulnerable on the outside was good for job interviews and attracting the wrong kind of men but a hindrance in so many other situations.

Warm water pounded inside my head, followed by the hard pressure of air. I lost track of the room around me as I spun at a speed never before reached. I flung my arms out in search of anything stable. Tears pooled on the inside rim of the goggles. The next wave of warm water slammed through my head, and the spinning room developed some sort of speed wobble. My mind ripped free, detached from the terror of the body in the way it must when the bear has you pinned, when the end is imminent and too terrible to watch.

"One more time," the tech said, and every muscle in my body tensed, and my mind bolted. Out of the claustrophobic room, away from the desperate city noise, back to the gray sheet of water stretching in front of my cabin, to the smooth, gray rocks under me as I lounged on the beach, the fire crackling next to me, crab pots soaking, rowboat waiting.

"That's it," he said, pulling the goggles off my face. "You can stay here for as long as you need to." He looked concerned. "Water?"

"No." I was curled up on my side, spitting into the bedpan, squinting at the corner of the room where the wall met the floor, trying to get it to stabilize. All I wanted was for him to go away.

"Well," he said. "It's good news at least. All the results are within normal range."

I was too tired to hate him. Too tired to say *Please stay*.

After he left I lay on the sticky paper, panting for a long time. The room stopped spinning but continued to slosh around me in an angry way. The need to be outside pressed down on me. I needed more air, more space. I slowly got to my feet and gathered up my things, keeping my head low.

I dragged a hand along the wall to be sure where it was as I made my way out a side door of the office that dropped me back in the hallway. The pictures on the walls became Medusa's hair. I put my hands on either side of my head like horse blinders and stumbled out, desperate for the icy wind.

Outside, I sat breathing for a minute with my back against the hard bricks of the building, knees drawn in like the fawn. Except she was on a pillow of snow in the deep woods, a creek running by. I was crouched on dirty snow, ugly buildings all around, indifferent cars driving by.

■ ■ ■

Late at night, in whispers.

ME: "You really should break up with me."

MIKE: "I don't want to break up with you."

ME: "This sucks for you."

MIKE: "It's worse for you."

ME: "You are the only peaceful place."

YEAR THREE

CHAPTER NINE

The acupuncturist who I was still seeing twice a week waited until the dizzy drain needles had been in for a while and the rest of me was loaded up with needles such that I couldn't move and pulled up a chair. "You know," she said, voice in butterscotch mode, "you can't control this illness."

I rolled my eyes over to her without moving my head. You can't control anything.

"But," she went on, picking through the words like someone in nice shoes on a muddy road, "you can control how long you spend feeling sorry for yourself."

The gauntlet thrown at my feet. In a nice, flowy skirted, Boulder way. She was right, of course. And she was wrong. But I loved her for sensing the railroad tracks, cool to the touch.

Her words stalked me like the ophthalmologist's. Always leaning up against a wall when I stepped out into a hallway, nudging me toward the obvious conclusion: While I could not control how sick I was or how sick I was to get, my agency crouched in the way I responded to it.

■ ■ ■

I dragged the yellow tape deck with the braille buttons out from under the bed. I put myself back in the fireproof suit and gloves, pulling my helmet on for a helicopter drop-off in the backcountry with a radio that only worked if there weren't too many mountains in the way. We control nothing. Bears charge, boats sink, we get left out overnight in wet clothes with no tent on uninhabited islands teeming with bears. We only have the ability to react. We can freak out and make the situation worse, or we can take a deep breath and calm down in the face of the calamity that was just as likely to happen as not. We can feel indignant that it happened to us, or we can just get on with dealing with it. I pressed play, told my mind that I liked listening to books, forced my brain to rearrange how it absorbed story until I was no longer a dizzy person curled up on a bed around a twelve-pound audiocassette player but instead was an Irish detective on the trail of the IRA.

■ ■ ■

On the internet, I learned Feldenkrais was a series of gentle physical exercises that can calm down and redirect your nervous system. Anything calming seemed like a good idea. The desperation stretched thin and taut like a piano string. I was willing to try anything.

There were a surprising number of practitioners to choose from within a ten-mile area. The first one I called laughed a little when I asked if she took insurance. The second one said no in a way that made me realize it wasn't worth calling the rest, so I went ahead and made an appointment.

She was an older woman with short gray hair and excessively soft hands. She led me back to a small yoga room with mats on the floor. She sat gracefully in the middle of the room and crossed her legs, so I followed suit. Her posture was perfect, and I tried to imitate it, divorcing myself of all logic, thinking that perhaps better posture was the first step toward getting my life back. She listened attentively to my long ass story, nodding, the dreadfulness of it gathering on her face. I wanted to hug her or have her hug me, I wasn't sure which.

"Do you think you can help?" I asked after concluding with the ENT torture chamber goggles. "Because nothing else has."

"I can try." She stood and offered me a hand, as if she were unsure I'd make it back to standing. She started with a few slow, balancing moves. I couldn't do any of them. The room moved and swayed and jumped, and I couldn't keep track of where the floor was. She moved from in front of me to behind me, her hands on my body, trying to help me keep things straight, but it was no use. I crumpled to the floor and waited on hands and knees for the room to calm itself down.

She rubbed my back in small, solid circles. "This isn't going to work for you."

On the way out, she refunded my credit card.

■ ■ ■

The rejections piled up. Seven, ten, eighteen, thirty-one. I read each one to Mike just to see what he would say. "She probably smells like cats. You don't want her for an agent."

At night, in the lab, I wrote with my eyes closed until the pen skidded against the desk, opened my eyes to line up right for the next line, and kept going. Mike typed them up in fifty-page batches. I gave Marta the broken-down barge that I once, in real life, wanted to buy to anchor off the shore of our cabin and use for a guest room. She dragged it out to a bay where everyone would leave her alone, anchored up, and got a dog.

I gave Jess all my own sadness but for a different reason, and she and Marta outwitted the institutional engine that is Smokey the Bear to actually save the trees.

I hauled my tape deck around and listened to stories when I got too dizzy to think. I plugged in earbuds and carried my twelve-pound four track player around the test center to endless jeers from the machinists and engineers I worked with:

"Maybe an iPod?"

"1983 called, they want their shit back."

Sounds mean, but it wasn't. It's not like I ever told any of them I was dizzy and I missed books like long ago sailors missed fruit. To them, I was just a bony girl who liked to trail fingers along walls and had an affinity for retro tape players.

I saw the acupuncturist twice a week, the young chiropractor with the red/green roller twice a week, and the cranial sacral lady twice a week. I spent as much time as I could in the rainforest with Jess and Marta, and in the world of any book I could get from the Library for the Blind. I moved from shadow to shadow, stayed hidden enough to stay out of reach of what was chasing me.

■ ■ ■

"Will you send me to Montana to learn how to climb trees?" I hovered in the door of my boss's office at the Forest Service in Alaska. He didn't like me. He was bald and moved too quick to keep good track of.

"Why would I do that?" He shuffled papers and didn't look up.

I held up the environmental impact statement for our forest, a document the Forest Service regularly put out for the public to know what we were doing to manage their land. "Because it says in here that we are monitoring for marbled murrelets and we're not."

Murrelets are small, squat, diving birds that partner for life and nest in old growth trees. If documented in an old growth stand, the Forest Service is supposed to protect that stand, or some portion of it, for the birds who depend on it. Problem is, murrelets are scrappy little birds that don't build nests. They hang out in the ocean all day with their significant other and then fly into the forest at night, selecting old growth trees with just the right amount of moss in the crook of a branch high up for a good night's rest. Since there is no evidence of a nest, it's hard to document them. You've got to climb using old school telephone pole climbing equipment that includes a big wide strap and spikes strapped onto your shoes. The Forest Service requires a class to be a certified climber. I'd found a class in Montana a few weeks out.

"And I'll need you to send Glen too. The Forest Service requires another certified climber on the ground if the first climber gets in trouble."

My boss gave me a flat look. But at least he'd stopped shuffling his papers. He took a deep breath of the stale air in his beige, cement block office. I knew I should stand up straight in front of his desk, demand in a clear way that the forest wasn't just for cutting down, but I remained slinked up against the doorframe.

His one leg began to jitter under the desk. If he said no, he'd be admitting that the environmental impact statement was a lie, but if he said yes and we started monitoring, we might find them, and that would jack up his proposed timber sales.

"Fine."

"Really?"

He squinted at me, so I left quickly. I thought of the spindly poles and how I would have on spikes and how it would be the same thing but based on fact instead of wild emotion.

■ ■ ■

The morning of our flight, I found Glen, the head of the wildlife crew, but he didn't look ready to head to the airport. I dropped my backpack on the floor of his office. "What's up?" I asked.

He leaned back in his chair and gripped either armrest. Our boss didn't like him either. "He canceled my trip."

"Did he cancel mine?"

"No. He says you can go now and I can go later."

I slumped into the extra chair in his office, beaten again by the powerful powers that be. "Murrelets have been documented flying fifty miles inland to find an old growth stand to bed down in. They're so small. They're diving birds." I'd been learning everything I could about them.

Glen cricked up one side of his mouth. "They have to flap so hard to keep their fat little bodies in the air. Makes you wonder why they sleep in the trees. Or why they can't just make do with the crappy second growth."

"Old growth has that good, billowy moss. I'd fly fifty miles if it got me to a Sleep Number bed instead of the crappy piece of foam on plywood I sleep on now."

He laughed.

"There's not another class until next summer." I pushed at my pack with my toe. "You think he'll send you then?"

"Not sure, but we'll keep asking."

I spent the next week in a surprisingly open, sunny forest in Missoula, climbing up to and beyond the seventy-five-foot mark to ensure I'd get hazard pay. "You're like a real grown-up on a business trip," a friend said. And I was, with my per diem and paid for hotel room. I congratulated myself that my business trip didn't include a single nice shirt.

I loved the weight of the strap, the clank of the harness, the timing of unweighting the strap to fling it higher up the trunk and then leaning against it to spike my feet higher. Up in the canopy, the wind took on a new sound unencumbered by the earth. There was the freedom of all that blue and so much room if only I could fly.

■　■　■

Late at night, in whispers.

> ME: "Do you think I feel sorry for myself?"
> MIKE: "Sometimes."

■ ■ ■

At the lab one evening, I rolled my chair over to the emergency exit door, pulled on my noise canceling headphones to block out the clicks and clacks of pointless aerospace, and watched the bare arms of the landscaped trees against the metal gray sky.

My favorite dive-bombing hawk was out there, pissed as usual. Perched in the highest branch of the highest tree, his yellow eye pinning me in place before he took off, deciding I wasn't worth it. Never mind the glass door between us. There were so many impossibilities in life. One more conversation with my dad. A day without dizziness.

I took a deep breath and tried noticing the smooth arc of the hawk's ever higher circles instead of the way my vision jumped and jerked him across the sky every half loop.

Maybe it was time to accept that I was no longer me. The idea of living with it was the equivalent of swallowing puked up puke, but maybe it was time. Maybe I could find a way of accepting this diminished version of myself.

Another engineer had the audacity to walk to his car, and the hawk pierced him with a look, dropped off his perch, and went for his head, talons out.

Or maybe, I thought as I watched the engineer hunch and run, I would just keep attacking the very idea of it.

■ ■ ■

On a day I knew I wasn't going to make it to Denver without causing a multicar pileup, I asked Mike to drive me down to an appointment. We were sitting at the table, him just returned from his forty-eight-hour shift, me having just dragged myself out of bed. He peered at me, likely trying to see what corner I'd turned that had led to the unusual request. I never really wanted to invite him into the sad display of my many appointments. It felt like some sort of wool shirt that I didn't relish him watching me squirm in.

"What time?" He worked at a busy station where all the firemen were medics. They often ran twenty or more medical calls in a shift and got about two or three hours of sleep a night.

"1:30."

"Wake me up at noon?" He leaned down to kiss me before he disappeared down the hall.

"Thanks."

I was constantly on the search for someone else who might be able to help, but this one today was a stretch and represented a whole new level of desperation. I was glad Mike didn't ask what kind of doctor he would be driving me to.

Later that afternoon, after he had tapped in the address I'd given him into his phone and I had white-knuckled the front seat of his truck all the way to Denver, we ended up at a tidy house in a run-down neighborhood.

"What's this?" he asked, peering through the passenger side window at the house, clearly expecting bricks and a sign out front directing us to the correct suite number.

"She's going to test me for hard metals. Freezers full of salmon, all those years . . ." I trailed off.

"At her house?"

"Yes." I was strung out so thin, I was sure he could see through me. All my desperation flapping in the wind.

"She's going to take the blood samples to a hospital?" Mike is a paramedic. He believes in science too.

"She's going to muscle test me."

He pressed his lips together. The wrinkles at the edges of his eyes deepened. "How's she do that?"

"By pressing on my arms." I opened my door. "I'll be done in an hour." I'd already had the blood tests looking for trace minerals and toxins. All clear. The logical part of me understood that toxins show up on blood tests taken at hospitals by people with gloves on. The tired part of me wondered if since the dizziness was elusive and unexplainable, then perhaps the cure was too. But I'd sound crazy if I said all that.

"Okay." Mike ran a hand down my back as I climbed out. "How much does she charge to press on your arms?"

My feet were on the ground, but I wasn't quite ready to let go my hold on the truck to walk the wide open distance of her driveway up to the front door. His judgment of my choices slapped like a wet rag. I looked up, wondering if this was the impasse we'd been heading toward all along.

But he was smiling. His grin like a point on the horizon where I could rest my seasick eyes. "'Cause I'll press on your arms for free."

I laughed, and the world righted itself for half a second.

The house was cluttered, and my eyes were doing the Alice in Wonderland thing where everything appeared much larger than I suspected it was and I felt much smaller than I knew I was.

The Chinese doctor who specialized in metals ushered me onto a narrow wooden chair in the center of her living room and settled herself on a matching chair, such that our knees were almost touching. I held various vials of heavy metals to my cheek while she pressed on my outstretched arm to determine any sensitivity. Sometimes my arm remained outstretched, and sometimes it gave under what seemed to be the exact same pressure from her. *Magical realism*, I thought. Aimee Bender, Karen Russell. Maybe you write about real things until unreal things start to happen in your life. Until what used to be straight and true no longer is and, suddenly, vampires live in lemon groves.

Each time my arm gave under her pressure, she held out a quick, efficient hand, and I gave her the vial that had just been up against my cheek. She checked the label and copied down the offending metal onto a sheet of paper balanced on her knees.

At the end, she had a long list.

"Well," she concluded, looking drained. "There is certainly a problem here."

"I ate a lot of salmon."

"I'll say." She breathed out heavily as she got to her feet. "I'll go mix up an herb formula that will help your body fight these contaminants." After she disappeared through a doorway, I stared at the ceramic angels on every available shelf in the living room, and I thought, *Maybe*. I thought, *Please*.

YEAR FOUR

CHAPTER TEN

The dive bombing hawk continued to assault engineers, techs, HR people on their way into work. I loved him. He was my hero. He screeched and came at anyone who annoyed him with talons flexed. I sat under florescent lights on sticky paper and took whatever came. "Okay," I said, "Okay." Over and over, when what I needed to do was rip up all the magazines, overturn the chairs, dive bomb their heads, set up a three legged perch across their parking lot, and strap on a bike helmet until we got somewhere.

■ ■ ■

The chiropractic integrative healer, who my aunt swore by, saw patients at her house up in the mountains on a horse property. An hour of her time was many hundreds of dollars, obviously not covered by any insurance. She greeted me at the oversized wooden door and asked me to take off my shoes. She was small and twiggy in the way of folks who do a lot of yoga and avoid gluten.

She led me through a main room with vaulted ceilings and a grand fireplace into a back room with a massage table. The window looked out over the horses in the field and the stacked up mountains in the distance, and I realized in the same moment that I wanted a view like this to call my own and that I would never have it, so long as the dizziness consumed my health and financial security in equal measure.

I didn't know what a chiropractic integrative healer was, but I hoped that she had somehow integrated her way out of the chiropractic side of things because I didn't have the stamina to withstand the violence of it after driving the twisty mountain road up to her house. She sat down on a chair across from me, all flat planes and sharp angles, alert and clear skinned from all the fruits and vegetables. The words I wanted eluded me, so I handed her my spreadsheet. She read every line and then tapped the table with two fingers and patted the massage table. "Let's take a look."

Once I lay down, she identified the there/possibly-not-there issue at C1 and jammed it back into correct alignment. She moved around the plates of my skull in the same way the other cranial sacral woman who typed in my insurance card numbers instead of my credit card number did twice a week. I fell into the same calm space cranial sacral work always created. And the minute she let go, I felt terrible again. Same, same. Except for the dollars.

"I'd like to muscle test again," she said as I lay there, the dizziness angry as that hawk, swooping back in, protecting its territory.

"Okay," I said.

"Elevated mercury levels. Too much salmon," she concluded a few minutes later.

"Yeah," I said. "That's what this lady said too." I pointed to line twenty-seven on the spreadsheet. "But I took the herbs and nothing changed."

She sighed a heavy sigh. "I'd like for you to try my herbs. They'll be quite different, I assure you."

My turn to sigh. Maybe the entire medical landscape was nothing more than the biggest corn maze ever created. Maybe all these doctors were just people, as lost as I was.

It seemed I had two options: wallow and give up, or push and get on with it. I leaned into the dizziness with my shoulder, dug my feet in, and threw all my weight into making room for me to live. I would Achieve Anyway.

With my new distinction of "visually handicapped," the state of Colorado required the university to convert any required reading materials for any class I took into audible files. Which was going to make it possible for me to reenroll in school, which seemed impossible, but I stayed focused on the idea that I would be able to fly my body not built for flying the long distance to get where I wanted to be. Somehow.

There was paperwork to drop off, so I drove over to campus. I found the Disability Service Office on campus but stalled out at the door. I stared at the stenciled word and felt it hovering over me. Was I disabled? I was limited, but disabled seems like a forever thing. This couldn't be a forever thing. Maybe this was going to be a forever thing. Fear crawled across every inch of my body as the hallway sloshed and swung underneath me. I tried to force myself across the last few steps to the doorway, but my feet wouldn't move. To walk through was to admit so much.

A smiley woman bustled up behind me, arms loaded down with files and papers. I was blocking her way, so she reached around me for the doorknob. "You coming in?" she said with a grace and ease that made it possible to say yes and follow her inside.

■ ■ ■

The aggressive grandma agent wrote to say she was giving up. After forty rejections from all the big and midsized presses, she'd run out of options. I sent her the first fifty pages of the Jess and Marta book and she wrote back:

i don't like this one.

It felt like I'd been clipped by a sharp arrow, but I kept running. Of course, the idea was to publish the books I was writing, but the more important thing was the refuge Marta's barge was. The way I could disappear into a world of my own making. The way I could feasibly persevere along with Jess and Marta as they got to the other side of all the struggles by the end of the book in a way I was not able to get to the other side of anything in my own life.

After six months, I gently broke up with the young chiropractor with the cold metal roller. There was artwork on every wall now, a plant in each corner. I poured alcohol in the wound by asking him who, in his opinion, was the best chiropractor in town. He squirmed a bit, but even he had to admit that despite all the red to green business, I wasn't getting any better.

He gave me a name and then said with a soft-shouldered wince, "But she's exorbitantly expensive."

Driving home, I decided, with distaste for myself and the world in general, I would try the expensive chiropractor, and then I would give up on C1 as the problem and on chiropractors altogether.

The expensive chiropractor was a runner. Something about the swishy ponytail and the protruding hip bones. The initial consultation was $800 and then $400 for each adjustment thereafter. No, she didn't like to bother with insurance. Took too much of her time.

With her cold roller, which I worked to convince myself was way different than the young guy's cold roller, she immediately identified the same issue with C1 and the occipital. I submitted myself and my credit card to biweekly appointments, which she suggested as the only possible treatment plan. At the conclusion of three months, with one last roller along my upper spine, she announced that C1 was back in place and holding. She was clearly proud of what she'd accomplished.

"But I'm still dizzy," I said. "Everyday." And my credit card is back in the four digits, I wanted to say but didn't. "The dizziness is as bad as ever."

She gave a tiny shrug, her shiny ponytail whipping as she hung the cold roller back on its holder. "Then I guess we know that C1 and the occipital aren't what's causing the dizziness." Like she was delivering good news. Like a cheerleader intent on being cheerful despite the scoreboard.

"Okay," I said. I wanted to kick her in the shins, ask for my thousands of dollars back, ask her if she enjoyed her ski-in, ski-out condo she'd bought by charging sick people incredible amounts of money. But I just walked out into the too bright parking lot, feeling like the desperate idiot I'd become.

■ ■ ■

I gave up trying to stave off the hot hatred of everything and everyone who felt fine. Instead, I let it consume me. I let myself actively hate anyone who was sick and got better, anyone who talked about their mountain biking weekend or walked their dog along the sidewalk as if the ground weren't moving. Anyone who complained about stupid shit. I let myself decide all shit was stupid.

Meanwhile, I went out to dinner with Mike and other couples. Stayed quiet, but I was quiet before I got sick and started hating everything. I made the right comments in the right places, contorted my face into smiles. I went to work, I went to class. I controlled chamber temperatures. I did not talk about dizziness or doctors or how everything was tinted red with the hate. The distance between how I seemed and how I actually was stretched to breaking.

■ ■ ■

I expected a call from the Center for Dizziness ENT texter to say, *Alright, well, since the air and water in your ear torture test came back normal, let's try this.* The call didn't come, so I called the office and asked if the doctor could call to follow-up and let me know what's next, given the test results.

"You'll need to make an appointment with him to discuss your care," said the receptionist.

"Couldn't he just—" I sighed. I knew he couldn't just.

"Let's see," he breathed. "Looks like the rest of this month and next month are all booked out."

The one-eyed drive down there was so long and those pictures in the hallway so awful. "Okay."

"His next available is July 28."

I wanted to explain that I might not make it another three months, that the railroad tracks were within walking distance. "Okay," I said.

He repeated the date and time and then added, "You'll need to be here one hour prior to the appointment for a hearing test."

"I don't need another hearing test, just an appointment."

"We hearing-test every single time."

"My insurance won't pay for it," I said as I watched a pencil on the desk in front of me move to some sort of staccato techno beat of my brain's making. "And the results were all normal. I'll consider another one possibly in the future, but nothing is going to change in three months. And those hearing tests aren't cheap." The receptionist remained huffy but allowed me to make an appointment without a hearing test.

Three months later, I one-eyed-pirated down the interstate and then horse-blinded my way down the hall and checked in at the front desk. "You're late," the receptionist behind the desk said in the same nasally, noncommittal tone he used on the phone. His shirt was tucked in very tight.

"My appointment is in forty-five minutes," I said, still reeling from the drive and the hallway and the PTSD of the torture goggles, now that I was back in the same space they were.

"Your hearing test was supposed to start fifteen minutes ago," he said.

"I don't need a hearing test. I'm here to see the doctor."

"You cannot be seen if you are late."

"I am not late. I have an appointment at 10:00. It's 9:15."

He breathed out loud through his nose. Leaned over to consult with someone I couldn't see off to his left in low whispers. I checked the height of the counter, vaguely registered that it wouldn't be that hard to climb over it and punch him in the throat. I stood there until he leaned back into my view. "Take a seat," he said.

Eventually, my name was called, and I was led to an exam room with a window that looked out over the parking lot. It was an unusually warm spring morning, and I was the first appointment of the day at 10:00 a.m. 10:15 slid by as I waited, then 10:30. At 10:45, the puffy faced doctor pulled into the parking lot below in his convertible Mercedes, sunglasses on, thin hair wisping in the wind.

He came through the exam room door ten minutes later in his white coat, fifty-five minutes past our scheduled appointment time.

"So," he said, settling on his rolly chair, staring into the computer screen. "Looks like all tests are normal."

So, I wanted to say, *you can be fifty-five minutes late, but I can't be forty-five minutes early? Why is your time more important than my time?* I wanted to ask him. Were you saving a life before you jumped into your convertible? Some sort of inner ear emergency across town? But I knew the answer. Because I am sick, I am lesser. Same in the animal world. Except there, once you become weak and mangled, you get eaten, and all the suffering ends.

■ ■ ■

"An outside wedding would be ideal," Mike said, his eyes alive with all the possibilities before us now that we'd decided to get married.

I poked at the eggs on my plate, trying to figure out how in the world I'd have enough energy to have relatives in the house who were bound to get hungry, how there were so many details of a wedding to keep track of, how I would walk around on uneven ground all day without falling over, how all I would remember of my wedding was how shitty I felt during it. "Let's elope."

His face fell, and I understood we would not elope. "But my family . . ." he started.

"I know," I said. All I wanted was for him to stay in my life forever. I couldn't imagine an existence without his humor, his arm around me, his kind, easy way. "Okay," I said.

■ ■ ■

It's not smart to hike in Alaska with a backpack full of bacon.

Elsie was in charge of the project. She was five feet tall and hit whatever she aimed her gun at. She had assembled an unlikely crew of international volunteers, Forest Service field crews, and Fish and Game employees to work together to help set

appropriate tag limits for bear hunters by setting 250 tetracycline bait boxes.

The idea was that the bears on the island would eat the anti-
biotic, which lays down a layer in bones that can been seen with
a black light. Fish and Game would ask hunters who killed a bear
on that particular island the following fall to turn in a toe bone,
which would be sent to Elsie. Based on how many were marked
by tetracycline and how many were not, she would determine
population size using an established formula of population
biologists.

I was part of the field team of six. We spent our first night on
the uninhabited island in the musty, cold garage of an abandoned
Forest Service logging camp, making the baits and cooking up the
fish juice. Elsie had picked up a couple rotting salmon at a nearby
stream and was boiling them in a dinged up soup pot over a Cole-
man stove.

We built balsa wood boxes, ten inches tall by six inches wide,
then stuffed them with four tetracycline pills wrapped in bacon.
We wedged in a bunch of meat scraps to snug it all up and then
nailed a top on. We piled up the finished bait boxes, which would
be placed throughout the island, one per square mile, over the
course of the next two weeks. Some by helicopter, some by truck,
most by foot.

My assigned field partner, Hans, and I set out the next morning, backpacks loaded up with packed bait boxes, extra bacon,
molasses, a spray bottle of rotten fish juice, a map, and six GPS
points where we were to hang bait boxes.

Our first set of GPS points led us to a partially logged, steep
hillside. I pulled over and shut off the faded orange, old Ford truck.

Rain splattered the windshield, making everything a dreary dark green color. "Ready?" I said, climbing out, wiping my hood up. The stuffed bait boxes knocked against each other as I shouldered my pack next to the truck.

Hans, thin, raincoated, and German, stepped around the front of the truck. He smacked his palms together and rubbed them furiously, either to warm up or work off some nervous energy for the stupidity that awaited us.

We followed the overgrown logging road on foot into a tunnel of dense alder shrub. The rain beat against the web of leaves over our heads as we climbed through the green archway, hunched over to fit through. "Smells like wet dog in here," I said in the dimness. This was usually the first indication a bear was close enough to be watching you. There wasn't much sunlight left after the thick cloud cover and the locked arms of alder branches over our heads. We both began searching for bears. In the pages of magazines, they look majestic. Up close, they smell disgusting.

Hans threw me a look, and his face dropped as his eyes landed on something over my shoulder. "Look at that," he said just barely above a whisper, pointing. There were four claw marks on the nearest branch, head high, deep, and freshly made. I slowly turned in a complete circle, looking for any sign of motion. Any brown in all the green. My hand dropped to the bear spray at my hip.

"I don't see anything," Hans whispered. Neither of us had a rifle. There were only so many, and we didn't have that far to go compared to other field groups.

"Me neither. Let's keep going," I said, my stomach filling with something sour.

The alder patch thinned and then ended. When the GPS said turn north, I looked up the tangled, steep hillside from the old logging road. "This way," I said and began pushing into the thick brush. We hiked a quarter mile in, dense blueberry shrub whipping us in the face, moss muffling our footsteps.

When the GPS said we were in the right spot, Hans pulled out a bait box and a couple nails. Elsie had instructed us to hang them on trees at head height—too high for wolves, just right for an upright six-foot black bear to grab with his mouth.

"No bear is going to find this one," Hans said, rain running down the sides of his face where it dripped off his hood. The bears mostly hung out down low at the streams, now that the salmon were in.

"Obviously, they pass through on the road." I flung my hand in the direction of the clawed up tree.

"They'll never find this bait."

"I'll make a trail." This had also been part of our instructions.

While Hans dug around his pack for a hammer, I started back the way we came, hanging strips of raw bacon on the shoulder high blueberry shrubs every couple feet, squirting fish juice on all the low plants, and trailing molasses on the forest floor, checking over my shoulder every five seconds, the sour pit in my stomach growing quickly into a knot.

The familiar buzz started up in my chest. The unpredictable situation demanding a hypervigilance that kept me poised and ready for the next Mrs. Jordan, who would place a gentle arm around me and say, *We've got to get to the hospital. Right now.*

As I double checked the tread on my boots for any trace of molasses and fish juice and obsessed over whether or not the rain had rinsed the smell of bacon off my rain gear, where I'd accidentally touched my thigh, I had an overwhelming sense of exhaustion. I suddenly didn't want to have to be on guard all the time. For the first time, I wondered if living this way was sustainable. But what choice did I have? Even when you thought you could relax, something was undoubtedly headed your way. Better to be ready for it. At least Alaska was honest about the way life worked.

I finished dribbling the molasses and draped the final piece of bacon from the pound I'd opened and double-bagged everything back into my pack, deciding I'd wait on the road for Hans to catch up. I ducked under the low branches of a dense line of trees and stepped onto the road right in front of a black bear.

His stomach bulged, ready for the coming winter, his legs were thick and powerful, his back wide and flat. He sniffed the air between us, dissecting my scent. I stood frozen, thirty feet separating us. He was at least four times larger than me.

I stopped breathing. There was nothing else moving. My world narrowed to the small patch of ground between me and the bear, to the way my heartbeat was closing up my throat. He stared directly into my eyes, which I kept averted.

He paced in a slow arc from one side of the road to the other, showing me his profile, the angle from which he looked the biggest.

This is the first stage of a fight in the bear world, to show your opponent how big you are.

I tried to back my way down the road, one slow step and then a second. He moved along with me. One step closer and then a second, still slowly walking his arc, still closing the distance.

I eased my pack off my shoulder, removing the can of bear spray from the outside pocket. He huffed and then clacked his teeth twice. Two signs of further agitation. Adrenaline piled up in my blood. He stood up on his back legs, which made him tower over me as I dropped my pack. Maybe it would keep him busy before he got to me.

He ignored the pack, sniffed the air, and dropped back down to continue his slow walk from one side of the road to the other, each time getting closer to me. The future narrowed to only one of two things, neither of which were my decision. He would let me be, or he would not. He kept his small, electric eyes focused on me as I did my best to avoid his while still watching him, to be ready when he charged.

My brain suddenly kicked back to life. It was telling me to bend down slowly, pick up a sharp rock at my foot, flip the top of the bear spray canister open.

When the bear was even with me, only six or seven feet away, he stopped and locked his eyes on my face. Long, slow minutes passed. I braced my feet. Tightened my grip on the rock and the bear spray. Ready. And not at all ready.

He swung his head in a slow swoop, and then his massive body followed as he turned and walked away with heavy, deliberate steps down the road without looking back once.

The adrenaline washed out into my legs, turning them numb. I slumped to the ground, wondering if I was strong enough to bend but not break under the constant pressure of Alaska's honesty.

■ ■ ■

Once the texter decided it wasn't my ears, I was sent on to the optometrist who worked with the Center for Dizziness. Even though everyone said it wasn't my eyes, it was my eyes. Everything continued to jump and jerk in my vision all day long.

After an extensive exam, he explained to me that my eyes were a symptom of the problem (whatever it was), not the problem itself. He prescribed dropping my prescription and wearing prism glasses to ease the strain on my eyes. Which sounded great, given that most days, by the afternoon, my eyes felt swollen in their sockets, hard to move. I ordered new contacts at the lower prescription and prism glasses. In the few weeks it took for the prism glasses to come in, I began to believe that they would enable me to ride in the car to look at wedding venues, to research wedding details online for longer than four minutes, to read. Every day, my grasp on the helium balloon of hope got sweatier.

I called the glasses store every day to see if my prism glasses had arrived yet. The woman patiently explained several times that she would call me when they were ready. She called on a Friday, too late for me to make it to the store before closing. All weekend I alternated between hope and dread that they would and wouldn't work.

"Want to come with me?" I asked Mike on Monday morning.

"To pick up the glasses?" he asked.

"Yeah." I imagined us going out for brunch afterward, me bespectacled, full of energy, not dizzy, excited about the wedding details instead of overwhelmed by them. Two people planning their future, instead of one constantly propping up the other.

"Sure." He smiled in a way that didn't look very much like a smile, likely sensing how all my eggs were in one basket teetering on the window ledge forty-two stories up.

I sat in a booth later, too sick to eat, the world blurry due to the decreased prescription, and the dizziness raging like a hurricane kicked up by the prism glasses. My head ached, and I wanted to sleep forever.

Mike picked up my hand where it lay limp next to the fork. "I'm sorry."

I looked at him. "I'm so tired."

"I know." He moved out of his side of the booth and into mine. Looped an arm around me. "We'll get through this." And I saw clearly what I'd been doing wrong. Hope isn't meant to be hung on prism glasses or men in white coats. It's meant to be hung on that two letter word, "we," spoken by someone who means it.

■ ■ ■

The vestibular physical therapist at the Center for Dizziness decided I had visual motion hypersensitivity. "We'll retrain your brain," she said. "You will learn how to be dizzy in the world," she said at our first meeting. "You'll need to come down to Denver twice a week for a couple months at the very least."

A week later, the drive to her PT center left me worn out enough to curl up on the sidewalk and sleep. I closed my eyes for one minute to rest and then stepped through darkened double doors into a big workout room full of torture contraptions for dizzy people.

"The idea is similar to allergy shots," she explained as she led me over to a modified treadmill. "We'll force, I like to say 'encourage,'" she said with a small smile, "your brain to get used to it. To not send floods of adrenaline through your veins at the slightest perceived motion of still surfaces." She tapped the handle of the treadmill. "Up you go."

The part you run on had been replaced with a round, flat surface that was still for a period of time, like a floor, and then would jerk unexpectedly one direction and then another, just like floors did. After the first two jerks, I doubled over on the railing, sure I was going to puke, uncertain where the floor was and where she was and where I was. I panted for a few minutes and then stood back up and gritted my teeth. Back in high school, allergy shots had rid me of the all winter long stuffed-up nose. It made sense, sort of. It seemed like it might work, sort of. The mind was a powerful place. I gave her a nod, and she hit go again.

Next, she had me stand on a square of thick, squishy foam. I didn't know I was falling until her strong arms were correcting me back to center. The world began to spiral away in the Alice in Wonderland way. The room got bigger as I got smaller until everything loomed over me. I crouched on the ground, spread my hands out as wide as they would go on the floor. This is still, I told myself. It's not moving. "Need a break?" she asked. A kind hand on my rounded back.

"Yeah," I whispered. Discomfort was a part of life. I knew this. I'd swallowed Alaska's lessons whole: I could sleep in wet sleeping bags on cold ground, or on the ice of glaciers, or in the arms of angry men. I could survive shipwrecks and homesteaders and falling through the ice. I could be cold and wet and shivering for hours, days, months. I could carry a pack almost as heavy as myself for miles, despite the blinding pain of an ankle with every step.

I closed my eyes on the blue plastic mat of the vestibular rehab center and told myself I could survive this too. Maybe that cold, hard coast had been a training ground for the indifference of the US medical system. Had pushed me to my limits so that I would know where they were and that we weren't there yet.

After some water in a chair in the corner, the vestibular PT closed me in a closet. The small, dark room enabled me to catch my breath. Until she turned on the disco ball. "Just for thirty seconds," the PT said. "You can take this one home. Thirty seconds every day for a week, then a minute each day of the following week, then we'll see how you're doing."

I immediately closed my eyes. There was no way I could watch swirling lights. What was she thinking? But what did I know? I wasn't employed by the Center for Dizziness. I hadn't put years of study into the field. I'd never heard of visual motion hypersensitivity. It sounded right. It also sounded like a diagnosis handed out by Captain Obvious. I left my body in the room with her and the disco ball and took off. Back to when life made sense. Back to when disco balls only had to do with fun nights out, too many beers, and a late night slice of pizza.

On my way out into the parking lot, I held the door for a girl my own age who lurched across the threshold using a cane. Dizziness was written in the squint of her eyes, the tension in her neck, the hand out to find the wall, and I saw clearly what I was heading toward. It would get worse. I would need a cane, I would have to give up my keys, my job, my book, my life. I rushed out to the car, afraid to see anything else, understanding clearly that the limit of what I could handle was within sight.

■ ■ ■

My days cleaved into two parts. All the minutes before the disco ball, in which I dreaded the thirty seconds of swirling lights, and all the minutes after the disco ball, in which the dizziness raged due to the swirling lights.

My teenage cousin threw the party he promised he wouldn't while house sitting for us. Because my brain didn't work right, I forgot which day we were coming back, and we came home a day earlier than I had told him. There were pizza boxes and beer cans everywhere, and in the middle of it all, the disco ball. I was mortified by this for some reason. It made me feel old, impossible to explain. Stretched out of reach from everyone.

Mike planned our wedding while I tried to get through every day. As he slept next to me one night, I watched the moonlight on the roof of the house next door, fear like a bird in my chest. I couldn't let Mike loop his life to mine. I wanted him to have something better, someone whole, a life less restrained. I curled up against his side, laid a hand on his chest, whispered, "Don't do it," to him or to me, I wasn't sure.

■ ■ ■

I craved the release of alcohol, the flood of ease that runs through the veins with a shot of whiskey, the loosening. I thought about it all the time, could almost taste it most of the time. When I gave in, the desired effect happened, a lightening of the soul so profound I felt almost happy for thirty minutes, sometimes only twenty. And then the dizziness came roaring back in, kicking mad, pulling me into depths so dark it was hard to find my way out.

■ ■ ■

The texting doctor ran out of ideas for me after the prism glasses and PT didn't fix me. I ignored his "there's nothing left for you" and scheduled my next appointment with his partner. I was still hooked by the name—the Center for Dizziness. Where else was I going to go?

The front desk guy and I settled into an uneasy agreement that I had to arrive thirty minutes prior to my appointment time with the doctor, even if I was going to refuse the hearing test.

On the morning of my first appointment with the texter's partner, there was a wreck and a huge backup on the highway. I rushed down the puke inducing hallway and burst into the waiting room. The receptionist guy shook his head. "You're too late."

I explained the traffic jam. "And besides, I'm still technically ten minutes early. My appointment isn't until 11:00, and you know I don't get the hearing test."

He shook his head again. "You'll have to reschedule." He tapped at his computer. "Her next available is in two months."

There were two other people in the waiting room. Old people. "You can't be serious," I said.

"October 28 at 3:00 p.m.?" he asked.

I wanted to roar, to climb over the desk and transfer all the dizziness and nausea and brain fog from my body to his with one huge electric zap arching from my hands into his pear shaped head. I wanted him to suffer. I wanted all of it to be over with. I slumped against the reception desk. The urge to beat up some skinny man who had nothing better to do with his life than taunt sick people drained out of me. I wanted to be in the woods. I wanted everything quiet.

■ ■ ■

On October 28 at 3:00 p.m., the texter's partner bustled into the room. I sat on the marginally reclined chair as she fired off questions and typed my answers into the computer, her back to me, my spreadsheet flung on the desk next to her. She asked about the dizziness in ways that forced one- or two-word answers.

"Yes," I said, dutifully. "No." Even though I had the sense that the answer actually lay buried in paragraphs.

She eventually spun around on the rolly chair. I wanted to talk more, sleuth out the answer. But it took so much effort just to get out the single syllables. She said, "You don't have visual motion hypersensitivity, but I'd like you to keep seeing the PT once a week just in case it begins to calm your symptoms down. You have dysautonomia."

"What do we do about that?"

"It's a disruption in the nervous system."

"Where in the nervous system?" I asked. "What is disrupted?"

She shrugged. "Hard to tell."

"So, basically, it's like saying someone is sad," I slouched back the chair. "There could be a thousand reasons why." The helium hope balloon instantly turned to concrete and settled on my chest.

She tilted her head one way, then the other, considering my analogy, making the wall behind her slosh. "Yes," she agreed before spinning back to her computer, making the room spin with her. "We'll start trying drugs, three-month trials until we find one that helps."

I was squinting into the bright florescent lights, trying to line up the words to say that I get all the side effects, that I was afraid of feeling any worse than I already did, that I was afraid of what I would do when the texter's partner hit the red button on the wall and a fluffy lady with strong perfume appeared. The texter's partner speed walked out of the room at the seven-minute mark.

I picked up the new drug at the pharmacy and shook one out into my hand in the car. Fear pulsed in my head underneath the headache. I squinted through the aggressive sun and watched the traffic on the road. So many people doing normal things, consumed with top layer worries, all the bottom layers clicking along as they should, unnoticed. I tried to convince myself that I would be one of those people again, concerned with work or future plans or where to go for dinner instead of how to survive this hour and the next one. I stared at the small pill in my hand and tried to convince myself that it would be okay. That it wouldn't hurl me into the scariest place I'd ever been. Minutes ticked by as I unscrewed the lid of the water bottle, turned the pill over in my hand. Tried to still the fear.

In the hours that followed, the dizziness turned hypercolored, kaleidoscoped around me, made it hard to move. I went to bed before the sun set and, a couple hours later, woke up to pee. I used the bed, and then the dresser, and then the wall, to make it to the bathroom. I slid down the wall as the bathroom spun and faded to black. I woke up in a pile of puke.

The next morning, I sat on hold for a long time, waiting for the texter's partner's medical assistant. "This drug is not going to work." I explained the puking and the blackout. "Can you ask the doctor to go ahead and prescribe whatever is next on the list to try?"

"You really should give it a three-month trial."

I had no idea what to say to that, so I just sat there.

"But if you feel you can't," she went on, "you'll just have to wait until your next appointment to see what the doctor thinks."

"My next appointment isn't for another three months. Can I just talk to her on the phone? It's a long drive, and that's a long time—"

"She doesn't consult with patients over the phone."

"We're just trialing a long list of drugs. There's really no consultation needed."

"You'll have to discuss this with her at your next appointment."

"Can you fit me in sooner, then?"

"She's booked up for the next three months."

YEAR FIVE

YEAR FIVE

CHAPTER ELEVEN

We spent forever trialing drugs. I got all the side effects that only 0.001 percent of people get. I turned into a real life version of that X-ray image, fragile and faded. More weight dropped off of me. I talked even less.

I tried each drug, suffered the three months until I could get in to see her again and report the drug had done nothing for the dizziness, only added numb limbs, a pounding heart that rattled my ribs and made me avoid ballparks, crippling constipation, all day diarrhea, insomnia, something similar to narcolepsy, etc.

Each time, the doctor consulted her computer, called in a new prescription, hit the red button on the wall, and the perfumed lady showed up to walk me out at the seven-minute mark. I began to covertly keep track of how many times she let me talk for longer than one to two sentences. Not once. But then she landed on Verapamil and I forgave her everything.

Within twenty-four hours of the first dose, the waterfall walls slowed to a trickle. The dense fog of my brain became a thin, steamy situation I could sort of see through. It was like someone had let me back on land. I still had the feeling of constant motion from the long sea journey, but it was subtler, the main mechanism removed.

The glorious pink and purple pill allowed me two pages of reading and seven or eight minutes at a time on the computer. I noticed for the first time how incredible the snowcapped mountains in the distance were, relished long walks in the open Colorado woods, held Mike's hand and laughed when he introduced me as his first wife to his fire chief.

In the late night clicking and clacking of aerospace, I learned to type with my eyes closed. It was the same drill, only peeking every so often to make sure things were still on track. I learned to slow down, to see every letter on an imagined screen in my head to decrease mistakes and stretch the seven or eight minutes of allotted screen time across an eight-hour shift. I marveled at how much faster work on the novel was without the writing in longhand step. Marta became a painter, Jess was mourning her inability to get pregnant. I was somewhere else for hours and hours at a time. And when I was in my own life, I just barely, barely started to think about a future in which I was better and Mike and I could make some decisions.

■ ■ ■

"What does it mean I have since the Verapamil works?" I asked the texter's partner, speaking fast because we were in minute six of seven and I knew she would reach for the red button soon.

She twisted up her mouth. "Verapamil affects many different systems in the body."

"Do you think I might stay stable enough to have a baby?" I asked.

Her eyes held mine for a minute. It was the first time I'd ever seen her completely still, stalled out for words. Weighted perhaps by the way I had become something more than a case sensitive to side effects. I had become a woman who wanted a baby. Minute seven ticked past and turned into minute eight. The bright overhead lights, the rolly chair, and the doctor coat fell away as boundaries dissolved. Me, the sad story, her tearing up. She cleared her throat. "That would be really hard, given your situation," she said, almost in slow motion, avoiding my eyes and reaching for the red button.

■　■　■

At my next appointment, my favorite front desk guy explained that the texter's partner had retired and that my appointment would be with her replacement. He turned out to be a man my height who had just graduated from Vanderbilt Med School. He was cocky in the way of boy-men who have finally found the respect they knew they deserved all along.

"There's no such diagnosis as dysautonomia," he told me straightaway. He chose to stand while I sat moderately reclined. He loomed over me, and I wished he'd sit on the rolly thing. "It's a nondiagnosis," he added. His hair had a lot of gel in it.

"What do you think I have, then?" I asked, sitting up straighter. I wanted to stand up, talk to him eye to eye, but I stayed where I was supposed to sit.

"Vestibular migraine."

Except that it wasn't vestibular migraine because the Topamax, from the doctor whose medical assistant had accused me of drug seeking, hadn't worked. But that all seemed like too many words to get out. I wondered if he'd read the spreadsheet in my file, where I had noted the previous vestibular migraine diagnosis and the fact that Topamax hadn't made the dizziness even incrementally better. I started to form the words, but he was barreling on.

"There's nothing more to do for vestibular migraine than take Verapamil. And since you are at the highest possible dose, this is as under control as it will ever be." He looked bored. "You should consider trying to decrease the amount of stress in your life."

■ ■ ■

That night, alone in the house because Mike was at the firehouse, the Vanderbilt doctor's words rang in my head. I went outside to get away from them, but they remained, loud and pounding, as I walked the sidewalks of the neighborhood. Life on Verapamil was better but only in the way running out of food was better than running out of water.

I lay down, thinking I'd fall asleep and that his words and that look on his face would go away, but instead, my chest tightened into a fist. I swallowed small sips of air, and the fist clamped down harder. Panic colored everything a deep purple in a way bears or weightless drops in planes never had. I rolled down to the floor next to the bed, air locked high up in my chest. On all fours, gasping like a fish on the bank, I knew for sure that if this was as good as it was ever going to be, then I was not going to last long.

Slowly, the panic eased and the sips of air became gulps. Mike's old yellow dog, Griffy, curled up next to me on the floor and we slept. The next morning, Griffy and I sat on the back deck. If this is the best it's going to be, can I be okay with that? I asked myself. The small hard pit of panic in my chest pulsed when I thought about it. Who wants to just survive minute after minute? Not me. Fishing or living in Maine or doing whatever my dead dad was doing while telling us he wasn't dead sounded much better. I shook my head to clear it. Who's to say I wouldn't be dizzy or otherwise mangled in that life too? And besides, Mike wouldn't be over there. And besides that, why do I trust the word of some guy who would undoubtedly get us killed in the backcountry if he was in charge out there? Because we are taught to trust doctors. We are taught they know more than us. But what does he know if he doesn't ask? What hidden pieces of the puzzle could he have possibly discovered in seven minutes of him talking at me?

"Alright," I whispered, the word puffing out into a cloud in the cold morning air. *You can control how long you spend feeling sorry for yourself.* "Alright," I said again, gathering up all the trust I had left in the world and placing it at the very center of myself. I would not accept that this was as good as it could get. I would keep searching for someone to help. I would do more than just survive. I would keep my head down, dig deep, and find a way to live anyway.

■ ■ ■

I convinced myself that I could live with discomfort. I shoved it into the corner of my mind, I ignored it, I endured it, I didn't talk about it. I stayed lost in the world of my novel as much as possible. The Verapamil cleaved off one whole arm of the dizziness, but it was super pissed and came at me from any angle it could find. I never knew when it would rage and when it would just sit and grumble in the corner, and so I lived in each moment like a crazed person. There was a volatility to it that I recognized. I kept still a lot, snuck around a lot, had a stomach full of slow burning fear that it would at any minute turn on me.

Jess and Marta beat the Forest Service at their own game, documenting old growth dependent marbled murrelets in the stand of trees they were trying to save.

I skipped the agent route and sent the book off to my favorite midsized press that accepted unagented work. Jess and Marta made the first cut, then the second. Eight hours at the lab without a book to work on felt like eighty-two, so I started a third book.

The fall before the dizziness and graduate school started, Karl and I had ridden the ferry twenty something hours to get to the road that led out of southeast Alaska to paddle the Yukon River for a couple weeks. There is often a Forest Service interpreter on the ferry to point out sea lion rookeries or passing whales. Karl was mad at me for the way I chewed or wore my shoes or something, so I had wandered off to the bow of the ship. It was a blue sky day, one of only a couple in southeast Alaska, and as we passed by an octagonal lighthouse in the middle of a narrow fjord, the Forest Service interpreter jumped on the intercom and said, "Hey, if anyone wants to live at that lighthouse, you can rent it for a dollar for a hundred years." And I thought, *Yes, that's what I'm going to do. That is the answer to all this. I'll be left alone in a beautiful place in an affordable way.*

After a couple weeks of paddling on the Yukon, we were back on the ferry. By then, it was mid to late August, which is basically winter, and the fjord was whipped up with screaming wind, and everything was gray and wet and scary looking. As we went by the lighthouse and the wind pushed at the concrete walls of it, I thought, *That is not the answer to this.*

But I couldn't get it out of my head. Surely someone would take the Coast Guard up on their offer. But who? And why? And what would it be like to live in the middle of the fjord alone without any way to get off the island except in calm weather?

■ ■ ■

In those late night hours, in between temperature readings, my fingers moved slow and purposeful and blind across the keyboard as I put myself back in southeast Alaska, moved out to a lighthouse with a not-so-great boyfriend who had secrets of his own. I walked the perimeter of the lighthouse island in the rubber boots of my character, unbothered by the sweep of the lighthouse light. I stayed up all hours with her as she smoked salmon and boiled water for a bath in a tub out in the yard. I cut wood and breathed in salt air and rested there at the water's edge in the shadow of sharp mountains.

I printed out the early drafts and memorized a paragraph at a time. Paced the concrete floors of the lab and repeated it over

204 Rachel Weaver

and over in my head, rearranging the words and the meaning until it lined up just right. Then back to the computer to type the new version of the single paragraph, fingers slow and precise, eyes squeezed tight. Some nights, I'd make it through two or three paragraphs, other nights only one. Some nights, I'd be too dizzy to do anything other than just think about what should happen out there in the channel, how my main character was going to deal with the next terrible thing I threw at her, and how she was going to overcome it. She was always going to overcome it.

It was so cold and desolate out at the lighthouse. The outside world matching my inside self. I slipped easily back into the life of my main character. I luxuriated in having a whole different set of problems whipped up by the wind and waves of coastal Alaska. For those hours, I was strong and capable. The wind was in my hair, and my shitty boyfriend was losing his mind from isolation. The humpbacks blew, and I had all evening in the glass top of the lighthouse to sketch the forever landscape.

Waiting rooms with fake waterfalls and bad magazines, cold, unwanted hands on my body, the anxiety of it all lasting forever, the news that my second novel was the last one cut from the final list at the midsized publishing house and would be joining my first novel in a drawer in the basement—all of it faded into nonexistence.

■ ■ ■

The dizziness eventually outsmarted the Verapamil. Some days, the Verapamil would get the upper hand, but mostly, the dizziness did whatever it wanted, and I suffered the consequences. I tricycle pedaled the rest of the way through graduate school. I visited the disabilities office each semester to drop off the books I needed converted to audio, I talked as little as possible in class to try to keep the room still. I drove to south Denver multiple times a month to the vestibular therapist who was working as hard as she could to retrain my brain how to live in the world dizzy. I hung up my diploma and stared at it. I tried to live in the world dizzy.

■ ■ ■

That night, skating under the moonlight, when the ice broke under me, I clawed and scraped at the edges of the ice to free myself. The icy water made it impossible to get a breath in or a scream out. And then, out of nowhere, my foot found purchase on a small shelf, and I launched myself out of the hole. I lay on the ice, panting, the jaws of Alaska having spit me back out, reminding me of all the things it had taught me so far: what we think is solid rarely is, life is full of discomfort, and sometimes, if you're lucky, there's a small shelf of land right where you need it to be.

YEAR SIX

CHAPTER TWELVE

Mike held my hand tight as we shuffled into the ultrasound room. He was jittery and couldn't stop smiling. We'd been seeing a midwife, and so the twenty-week ultrasound would be our first. My stomach had expanded rapidly, along with Mike's joy.

I lay down on the exam table, and the ultrasound tech turned off the overhead lights. "Okay," she said, looking over our file, her hair still shiny in the low light. "So you've not seen the baby yet?"

"No," I croaked out, dreading the news of a messed up baby growing in my messed up body. What if it was born dizzy? The thought snapped like a live wire in my chest.

She spread jelly over my enormous belly and ran the wand thing over it. The large screen in front of us lit up with a ghost image I couldn't make sense of. It was blurry and disjointed, and I was sure I was about to receive the news that I'd grown a baby who would have to live with some permanent, awful condition. I closed my eyes.

"So," she began, angling the wand far over to the right of my belly. "Here's the spine . . ."

Eyes still closed, I felt a small bit of solace in the fact that she hadn't gasped or let go an *oh god* as she studied the image. I took a peek, and my breath caught as a foreign sensation bubbled high in my chest. It took a minute to land on what it was. Happiness. I felt happy enough to chase out all the rest of everything for the first time in years. I held tight to it like a drowning person.

"And here's the head . . ." the tech was saying, and I could see it, emerging out of the haze on the screen. I glanced over at Mike where he sat on the other side of me, still holding my hand. He was as riveted as I was, eyes wide, taking in every bit of the hazy glow that was our baby.

"And here's . . ." the tech faltered. She peered at the screen and tilted her head. I felt like I was falling. I gripped the bed under me, braced for the news of some horrible abnormality that would forever limit the life I had just been imagining for the small being swimming around in my belly. ". . . the other baby," she concluded.

"What!?" Mike yelled, dropping my hand to step as close to the screen as he could get. "Where?"

I was up on my elbows, breathing hard to catch up. There were no twins in either of our families. Mike and I hadn't had any sort of fertility treatments.

"That's a really funny ultrasound joke, right?" I tossed her a half smile. She was standing up now, moving her wand, squinting into the screen in front of her. "There's only one baby," I said to set her straight.

"No," she looked at me. "You are definitely having two babies. I'm just looking to see if there's a third."

"We're going to need a bigger car," Mike said, turning toward me, pale and wide-eyed.

I couldn't take my eyes off the screen. Three babies. Holy mother of fuck.

"Okay," she sighed. "Looks like two healthy baby boys. Congratulations. Let me go get the doctor." She bustled out of the room, and I collapsed on the crinkly paper, my stomach huge and looming.

"They're healthy," I said to Mike in the dim silence of the room, the word looping around me like a life preserver. "And there's only two."

"Two!" he repeated. "Holy shit!"

The doctor who came in explained that the babies' heartbeats had been synced each time the midwives had listened with the Doppler at our previous appointments. I had not been gaining any more weight than a singleton pregnancy because of the severe morning sickness that had a dumb name because it was not limited to the morning. The doctor went on to explain that it was now considered a high risk pregnancy and my days with the soothing midwives were over.

Mike and I lay in bed that night in a stunned amazement. Mike trying to get used to the idea of twins, me holding onto the word "healthy." Repeating it over and over. They could be healthy even if I was not. They would be okay.

■ ■ ■

The phone rang. I was on bed rest because I had gone into labor at thirty weeks. I had been instructed to get up only to go to the bathroom and to shower. "No making yourself even a single piece of toast," the OB had said.

We unfolded the foldaway couch bed so I could hang out in the living room, which was great when Mike was around and lonely when he was not. He would pack up the cooler next to me with food and fill up several water bottles and leave me alone for forty-eight hours. My brother, who had moved to Denver by then, would come over after work sometimes and cook me alarming amounts of sausage that I would devour. You'd think you'd get a lot of stuff done or that laying around in bed all day would be relaxing, but neither of these things proved true. I watched my neighbors through the front window and worried about babies born too early.

So, when the phone rang, I was going to talk to whoever it was, even if they were going to try to sell me siding. "Hello?" I said.

"Is this Rachel?" a woman's voice asked.

"Yes," I said, my cheeks weird and swollen up with all the water retention.

"This is Susan Ramer. I just read your novel. I absolutely loved it."

"You what?"

"I'd like to offer you representation."

"What?!" I said again and then searched the recesses of my mind to try to come up with some other words to say. I had all but given up on any agents wanting my book after racking up a tower of rejections. "Yes! Holy shit! Yes!" I tried to sit up but that was not possible. "Sorry for the cussing," I added.

She laughed. "The book needs some big, overhaul type revisions. Are you willing to do that? And do you have the time?"

"Yes. Absolutely." I knew two things for certain: I shouldn't tell her I was about to have two babies, and I shouldn't mention that I couldn't look at a computer screen for more than eight consecutive minutes.

"Okay, well, I'll email over a contract with my editorial comments today. Give me a call when you've had a chance to read through it all and we'll take it from there."

After we got off the phone, I wrapped my whale body around Roxy Lou, who joined us after Griffy gave up the good fight at eighteen years old. Rox was a pound dog who thought the folded out couch was fantastic, and she could be found lounging at my side at all times. She accepted my hug with a groan sigh. We lay nose to nose for some time while I glowed. "I did it, Rox," I told her more than once. "I did it." As I lay there, I could feel the cold concrete of the lab under my feet as I paced through all those long, dark hours, memorizing the novel line by line. Rearranged it while it rearranged me.

■ ■ ■

I stayed on the lower dose of Verapamil in the early months of the boys' lives under the false pretext that good mothers don't give their babies formula. Two months into my new life with two infants and very little sleep, the dizziness raged free of any constraints. Walls went back to sloshing, and floors slid around. My stomach remained tight and up at the back of my throat, threatening to reject any food I attempted to eat. The boys were born four and a half hours apart; I hemorrhaged and was unconscious for the first twelve hours of their lives. The loss of blood left me too weak to stand up in the shower long enough to both shampoo *and* condition for months. I settled on shampoo only when there was time to take a shower, which wasn't often.

There was no one to help in the all-the-time way I needed it. Mike went back to working forty-eight-hour shifts. By the time one baby had been fed, supplemented, rocked to sleep, the other was ready to have his diaper changed, be fed, supplemented, then rocked to sleep. Twenty minutes later, the first was ready again. Babies are meant to be held. I tried to hold one while attending to the other, but that usually ended up in both crying. And so I settled for leaving one to cry while I fed/diapered/burped/bounced to sleep the other one. The world filled up with unmet needs, mine and theirs, pounding in my head, along my veins, into my heart.

They needed so much, and I had nothing left to give as my body worked to replace the blood I'd lost, to find some semblance of balance in the blind rage of the dizziness.

It was the first thing in my life that I knew for sure I couldn't do.

I needed to sleep.

I needed quiet to bring the dizziness under control.

Instead, I stayed awake, changed diapers, fed and rocked babies, mourned over some image I'd had of a mother in a rocking chair in the quiet, dim light of early morning, breastfeeding her infant, gazing lovingly at his every feature.

Fear choked me. There was no way through and no way out. I would fail them.

I pushed so hard against the exhaustion and the dizziness that the world began to feel unreal. As though I were floating through some warped Technicolor version of it. As though it had nothing to do with me and I had nothing to do with it.

■ ■ ■

The vestibular PT continued trying to break my brain and teach it a new normal, like a wild horse. When the boys were three or four months old, she found me sobbing in the small, dark closet where I was supposed to be staring at a piece of tape on the wall while the disco ball whirled lights past. I had held it together for so long. Something about the small, dark space, the way I'd been shredded down to nothing. It all caught up to me. She bustled into the room and closed the door behind her. "Oh no," she said. She was a kind, momish lady who I was sure breastfed her children and held them and didn't leave them crying on the floor until their faces turned purple while she tried to get the other one to latch on.

I couldn't stop crying. There was so much to cry about. She squatted next to me, one hand on my knee, the other on my shoulder, and gave me all the time and space I needed.

As I vaguely began to pull myself together, she said, "I heard about an allergist in town who has had some success with dizzy patients."

I couldn't imagine trying to explain the whole story to one more person. To sit in one more doctor's office. To watch one more person tap at a computer and ask me if I ever smoked. But I liked the PT and couldn't yet talk, so I just nodded.

She left me alone, closing the door behind her to leave me in the dark instead of leading me back out into the overly lit world, a small kindness that made me cry harder. She eventually returned with a box of Kleenex and the allergist's name and number.

■ ■ ■

The allergist looked like everyone's favorite grandpa. He had the tangly beard and the belly, the noisy breathing and the twinkly eyes. He invited me into his office, which was not an exam room but an actual office with a messy desk and pictures of grandkids everywhere. There was one of him dressed up like Santa.

He sat in his chair and motioned me to the other. He laced his fingers over the ridge of his stomach and asked me to tell him the story. I got the distinct impression that the PT had called him and said something along the lines of, *This one is fragile.*

I sat in the seat he'd indicated, which put us eye to eye. It was a small office with a desk against a wall. He'd turned his chair away from the desk so we were only a few feet apart. He smiled, and I took a deep breath. There was no fluorescent light or sticky paper, which made it easier to utter the first few worn out sentences of the story. I stopped where I was usually interrupted, but he just nodded, waited. So I kept going. The long list of doctors and diagnoses, the tests and blood work and small, thin needles, the hands that I allowed to manipulate bone. He listened and watched me, nodding here and there.

When I came to the end of the saga, he asked a few pointed questions about history of allergy.

"Yes," I said. "Tons of allergies as a kid. In high school and college, I had the shots."

"How long ago was that?" he asked. "How often do you feel as though you are having an allergic reaction to something?" He didn't write anything down, just listened, ignored his computer. I was worn out by hope, but it crept back in as he asked more questions, gathered various pieces of the puzzle, worked at fitting them together this way and that in his mind.

Somewhere around the forty-five-minute mark, he said, "I suspect you have a fair amount of inflammation from histamines that may be adding to or causing the dizziness. Allergy shots typically only last ten to fifteen years, and it's been what?"

"Fifteen," I said.

"Ah," he smiled. "Let's try a steroid."

I drove straight to the pharmacy, waited while the prescription was filled, and took the small, white pill in the parking lot before the fear of it could get me by the throat.

Within days, the walls stopped shimmering. Floors stopped rippling. Lamps stopped hovering, unsteady on desks. I did everything else the allergist suggested: ran the HVAC system in the house on fan only in the middle of summer, vacuumed up a bag of dust and sent it off to Johns Hopkins to identify the exact allergens in my house.

I filled three more prescriptions he ordered and bought an old person's pill container with MTWTFSS in big bold letters on each pop lid to keep them all straight.

For the first time, I found the joy that hid beneath the tasks of motherhood. I delighted in Wes's soft skin against my own, the look of intense concentration on Nate's face as he swung his arms in wild abandon at a crinkly elephant I made dance in front of him. I cried at the miracle of them sleeping together in their crib, instead of for my own misfortune.

The dizziness remained, a beehive in my chest, constantly humming, but the MTWTFSS pills allowed me to catch my breath, to become aware of other things besides bees buzzing.

After a month's long breath, everything stopped working. The dizziness blew back in like a Wyoming wind. I had to hold onto the dresser, then the wall, then the crib to get to the babies when they cried in the night. All day, every day, I remained in a dizzy stupor. The knowledge that I could not take care of myself or my babies in the way I knew I needed to closed over my head like the lid of a tomb. The knowledge that I might never be free of it dropped on top like loose earth.

I needed to sleep. I needed to find a doctor to figure this out. I needed to look at the train schedule. But instead, I washed bottles, changed diapers, made dinner, folded onesies, and matched socks. Got up at all hours of the night, held crying babies, and dug as deep as I'd ever dug for the willpower necessary to get through.

Between staying up all night at work, managing a sick wife and two infants, Mike took on the look of the walking dead.

■ ■ ■

The allergist was stumped. My allergy tests came back showing I was allergic to most things. He arranged for me to get allergy shots close to home so that I could bring the babies with me when

Mike was at work. But each time I got the shots, I was set to spinning and had to lay down in the hallway or in the car until I could drive the three of us home.

"We have to stop the allergy shots," the allergist said a few weeks later. We sat in his office with his pictures all around. "You can't accomplish what you need to if we are flaring up the dizziness twice a week."

I just looked at him. The end of another road was too much.

He fixed me with a concerned look, all bushy eyebrows and kind grandpa eyes. "I have an old friend, a very good doctor, retired now, but his son is an ENT over at the hospital. A very smart man. Histamines are part of the problem, but I'm convinced they aren't the source of the problem. Perhaps you have something going on in your inner ear that is hard to detect and will take a very specific mind."

Because I trusted the allergist and actually wished he was my grandpa, I agreed to try one last ENT.

■　■　■

Mike was a genius with babies. When he was home for his four-day stretches, he would take over to create blocks of time in which I could work on all the revisions Susan was asking for. My fancy skill of typing with my eyes closed wasn't much help in the face of revisions. I printed everything out and made notes in the margins. I crossed out huge sections and wrote replacement chapters longhand on yellow lined paper. I would take over the babies, and Mike would enter the revisions into the Word document, saving me from the dreaded screen time. His shoulders hunched over my computer caught me one afternoon as I fed pureed squash to the boys. A solid sign of love in an unsteady world.

I finished the revisions and sent the book back to Susan. I opened her response email with both fussy kids in my lap, one on each knee, computer on a jumble of mail on the kitchen table.

She told me in a kind, detailed way what I had suspected but had not been able to admit to myself. I'd moved things around but had just barely scratched the surface of the issues at the heart of the novel that still remained. I felt certain I did not have the bandwidth to do what needed to be done.

I cried. The boys cried.

I still hadn't come clean about having babies. How to tell her that it was impossible to hold enough thoughts in my mind at once to get beyond the surface of anything? I felt the need to apologize to that younger me who launched out of Alaska, driven by this dream I had just crashed into the side of a mountain.

I felt sorry for myself for two weeks, and then I wrote her back:

Dear Susan,

Can I have one more chance? I'll need eight months.

Dear Rachel,

Yes. Looking forward to reading it.

■ ■ ■

One thing I'd noticed about Mike over the years was that he was his most creative after three beers. I found a babysitter and told him we were going on a date. We walked downtown, and I waited until the magic three-beer mark. We sat at a high -top bar table in a darkened room with red walls. "Alright," I said, our knees all mixed up under the table. Mike looked alarmed, clearly unaware the evening had an agenda. "The problem with the novel is the middle," I said. "It's boring. The tension leaks out. I need something big to happen to disrupt everything."

Mike shot me a wild eyed look. I'd never asked him to help me with the book in this way. He'd just been promoted from secretary to VP and he knew it. "Okay," he said, adjusting in his chair and squinting up one eye. "I got it."

"You got it?" I asked. "Already?"

He was nodding. "What if William Harris is Kyle's dad?" He was still nodding, a huge grin spreading across his face.

"He's not his dad." I said. That would screw up everything from page seventeen to 245.

"But what if he was?" Mike smacked the table. "What if he was?"

"Shit." All the jagged edges of the plot were clicking together like puzzle pieces in my mind. It would solve everything. And it would mean starting over.

■　■　■

The last ENT had huge, rounded shoulders like a brown bear. He entered the exam room in a hurry, the sides of his white coat flapping. "Hello," he nodded to me as he sat in the rolly chair and sidled up next to the computer. I handed him my spreadsheet that had gotten a little sweaty in my hand while I'd waited. "Here's everything," I said.

He glanced at the first of the four pages and set it aside to focus back on the computer. He began to ask me the yes/no questions.

This was going to take so much more than monosyllables, but I went ahead and answered. "Yes," I said. "No."

He filled in the final field on the computer, then flipped through the final four sheets of my spreadsheet faster than the fastest speed reader alive, and then looked at me for the first time. "There's one option that hasn't been explored," he said.

I could barely swallow. *Please, please, please solve this*, I wanted to beg. The words pounded through my head, filling up all the space, vacuuming up any room left for any sort of response.

He turned back to the computer. "I'm going to order an MRI." His big fingers tapped at the keys.

My heart sank. He sucked at speed reading. "Did you see, there?" I pointed to the spreadsheet. "I've had two."

"This one will be a bit different. I suspect you have an operable condition in your inner ear. But in order to see if I can operate, you'll need to have a very specific type of MRI. And I'll have to be the one to read it."

He hit enter and stood up to leave in one quick motion. "The receptionist will give you the details on the MRI. It'll take a month or so to get on their schedule, and then you can schedule a follow-up with me." He was halfway out the door.

I looked at his hands. Was I going to let those hands cut into my head? Fish around my inner ear? We'd spent five and a half minutes together.

"Okay," I said.

I folded up the paper the receptionist gave me on my way out explaining who to call and where to go for the special MRI. Back in the hallway outside his office, I had no idea which way to go to get out. Always in search of the stairs because elevators aren't for dizzy people, my path to locating offices in multistoried buildings typically involved a long series of hallways to find the stairs and then a lot of wandering around once I was on the correct floor. I glanced down the hallway in one direction, and the patterned carpet got me. I closed my eyes to stop the spin, and the dark felt good. I sat down in the hallway with my back up against the wall. I needed a minute anyway to consider the idea of letting someone cut open my head. How do you operate on the inner ear anyway? Isn't it a closed system like a grape that, once popped, won't go back together? Wasn't I worth an explanation?

I was not.

But I didn't care. I was breathless at the idea that a surgery could fix me. When I opened my eyes, I noticed the migraine clinic across the hall. I flashed back to the confident look on Vanderbilt's face as he explained there was nothing left to do. Take that, Vandy. An operable condition. There was something to do, after all.

I stood up, found the stairs eventually, and ended up on the hard concrete of Denver. Yes, I decided, I'd let him cut open my head. What did I have to lose? If there was a chance it would stop the spinning, then yes, go ahead, strange bear man, make it worse or better. Just do something.

■ ■ ■

Two months later, after I'd been worked into the special MRI schedule and the results were in and the doctor had finally reviewed them, his nurse called to schedule me an appointment to discuss the results and possible impending surgery.

"I know you aren't able to tell me the results of the MRI over the phone," I said.

"Right," she agreed.

"But if we are going to discuss cutting open my head, I'd like to have my husband there. I don't always catch all the details when I start to get scared."

The nurse didn't say anything, so I barreled on. "We're broke . . ." I trailed off. Swallowed. Forced myself on. "If my husband comes with me, I have to find a sitter for my kids, which I don't want to do if the doctor is just going to tell me the MRI came back normal and there's nothing he can do. Can you just tell me if I should get a sitter?"

In the long pause that followed, I imagined that she got it. That she had kids too, that she was familiar with the financial burden of childcare. "You should get a sitter," she said.

I took his first available appointment, which landed us in rush hour traffic. Despite the hour and a half in bumper to bumper traffic, hope had me in a frenzy.

All I could think about was waking up in a starched clean hospital room Not Dizzy. Emerging. Back into life. Playing with the boys, rolling around with them on the carpet. I imagined having enough energy to pack up and take them camping one day. I was more talkative than normal, and Mike kept glancing my way, pleased or possibly scared out of his mind.

We settled into the exam room. It was small and white and cold, like all of them, but I hardly noticed. Hope kept me upright, alert. When the ENT walked in, his eyes immediately jumped to Mike. The doctor straightened to his full height and held out a hand. I tried to remember any doctor offering me a hand to shake and came up with one, maybe two, in the past thirty something. Mike and the doctor met each other eye to eye and nodded. They shook with a firm grip. I remained seated. What the actual fuck.

The doctor sat on the rolly chair. "The MRI shows a slight abnormality in the inner ear," he said, and I knew I'd made it. I'd survived all of it to get to this point, this person, who had finally, finally found the answer. "But it's fairly common, and it doesn't cause dizziness." His words slammed up toward me like concrete when you jump off a roof.

Me camping with the boys slipped away. As did skiing. And any sort of future. "There's nothing wrong with you," he concluded, getting to his feet. He nodded to Mike again, opened the door, and left.

On the way out, because I was terrified, I walked into the migraine clinic across the hallway. If two different doctors had concluded vestibular migraine, maybe there was something to it. If I had an appointment scheduled, there was still a flicker of hope. I would not do what I was afraid I'd do. Instead, I'd show up at the appointment.

The migraine doctor's next available was three months out.

I cried silently as we drove home. Mike held my hand the whole way. I knew the migraine doctor would be like all the others. She would incline her head, her eyes would glaze over, she would tell me there really was nothing wrong. It was over. But how to cut free the three people tethered to me?

■ ■ ■

I moved through daily tasks in a stupor, the dizziness huge and looming with sharp teeth and wild eyes. The world and all the people in it were so far away, even if they were right there. Often, I watched myself from up above myself. I spent a lot of time wondering who that person was shopping at the Super Target or buzzing up carrots, how she was managing all these impossible tasks. Wondering what would happen when she finally crumpled.

In the days before the first appointment at the migraine clinic, I didn't feel hope. I only felt numb.

The migraine doctor across the hall was so thin, she looked vacuum-sealed. Her short hair swiped along one side and spiked up a few inches on the other.

She pressed her lips together as she looked over my half-assed attempt at filling out the mountain of paperwork I'd been handed in the waiting room. The dizziness had its fingers dug so deeply into me after the long drive that I could only read in small snippets, so I tried to answer what I thought was most pertinent.

"Here's a spreadsheet of all the doctors I've seen and the diagnoses I've been given."

She studied every line of it with the intensity I imagined she brought to every mile of a marathon.

I waited until she looked up, nervous because we'd already used up three minutes. "I'm hoping you can weigh in on whether or not you think it's vestibular migraine."

She shook her head quickly, as if shaking off a bad smell. "Do you see auras?" she asked.

"No."

"How bad are the headaches?"

"I've had a headache for years, but it's not blinding like migraine is supposed to be. It's more annoying than painful," I said.

"Does Advil get rid of it?" she asked, facing the computer screen, typing faster than most fiction writers. "Is it only on one side?"

"Not really."

She handed over a sheet of paper with grid lines and impossibly small words that jerked and jumped all over the page. "This is a headache journal. I want you to keep track of every day. You'll need to note everything: your menstrual cycle, exactly what you eat throughout the day, exact time you wake up and go to sleep, all activities throughout the day, the weather, your bowel movements, and the severity of the headache."

I looked at the graph, tried to decipher the two-millimeter squares I was supposed to fill in. I didn't even have time to brush my teeth most days. The lines snaked across the page, and the room lifted up as if we'd just gone over a big roller. I stared at the corner of the room and took a breath to try to still the motion of everything around me.

"Do you mean the severity of the dizziness? The headache is really pretty much the same all the time," I explained. "Can we just talk it through? Or can I write out when the dizziness changes on something unlined? I can't really look at this." I waved my hand over the paper. "It stirs up the dizziness something awful."

"Doesn't sound like migraine," she said. "But we can do a few drug trials to see if anything helps."

She stood up. "My PA will be in shortly." She turned back just before she slipped out the door. "If you can't keep a headache journal, it's going to be very hard to treat you. All the information I need is on that sheet of paper."

I nodded, folded it up so that the lines didn't catch my eye, and slid it into my back pocket, still unsure if she wanted me to track the headache or the dizziness. Easy enough really, both were all the time. I'd just color in the whole fucking sheet.

She closed the door, and I slouched in the chair. Why are all dizzy doctors in south Denver? The drive was too much, talking to her was too much, her headache journal was too much.

I was still slouched in the chair, about to nod off, when the PA walked in. She was my age, had a bit of a haggard look and a long, printed out list of drugs. She sat down and looked at me for longer than a second. Saw me. Her face creased. "Is it bad today?"

This simple kindness let loose the tears. "I'm sorry," I said, wiping my nose on my sleeve. "I didn't mean to . . ."

She smiled. Found some Kleenex. "It's okay. I cry like that and I don't even have migraines. All I've got is a three-year-old."

"I have one-year-old twins," I blubbered.

"Oh god," she said, eyes wide. "I cannot imagine that." She shook her head, noticed the list still gripped in her hand. "The doctor wants to start at the top, but I brought this list in so you can see how many more there are to try if this first one doesn't work."

She set the list on the edge of the desk between us. "All these are used to treat vestibular migraine?" I asked. There were at least fifty drugs in all their capitalized glory. "Not just Topamax and Verapamil?" I wanted to wallpaper the house with it, drive over to Dr. Vanderbilt, and shove the list into his chest. I suddenly loved the ultramarathoner and this PA.

She laughed a little, thinking I'd made a joke. "We treat migraine with a lot more than Topamax and Verapamil. I'll just put a little star here next to those so we know they've already been tried." She drew a perfect star, like a mom of a three-year-old who spent lazy afternoons coloring, adding stars to the unicorn's eyes.

"Vestibular migraine?" I tried to clarify again.

She looked up. "These are all migraine drugs. I don't know much about vestibular migraine in particular, but I'll find out. I'm new here," she added.

I stared at the sheet. A whole page of options. Maybe. If vestibular migraine and migraine were the same thing. The myriad of tortuous side effects would be worth it to find the one magic pill that would work. "Thank you," I whispered.

"Of course," she said, her eyes all crinkled up in a smile. "We'll figure it out."

YEAR SEVEN

CHAPTER THIRTEEN

That "we" kept my head above water. Through ballooning bowels, through the inability to stay awake, the inability to sleep, the inability to drink enough water to quench a thirst wider than a red, crusty desert. Through months of a stomach that refused food, through hanging on by my fingernails for three months until my next appointment, when I could report that some drugs did nothing, some took the sharp edge off the dizziness, some made it worse, and none got rid of it.

I was not allowed to come back any earlier than three months after my last visit. The doctor was busy and booked that far out, it was explained to me by the bubbly, migraine free receptionist. Some drugs were too miserable to make it through a full week, much less the suggested three-month trial. But I had to wait until my next appointment, always.

The migraine doctor got progressively more annoyed at my monthly headache diaries. I tried, but to sort out the grid and follow the lines to fill in the correct four-millimeter square cost me so many dizzy dollars. And invariably, every time I sat down to try, the boys would cry or scream, or something would crash down and I'd be interrupted. Three days later, I'd get back to it and try to remember if I'd woken up four or five times three nights ago. My last period might've been the decade before, maybe I had eaten a bag of M&M's on Tuesday or Saturday. The migraine doctor wanted data. If there was no data to pore over, there was nothing to talk about. She spent six minutes in the room every three months and prescribed a different medication from the list that was gaining unicorn stars at an alarming rate.

"Can this just happen over the phone?" I asked at one visit, sure I would careen off the highway sooner or later driving down to her office.

"No."

■ ■ ■

Every three months, a new drug. Every three months, a new side effect.

The aerospace lab hired me back, agreed to let me work only on the days Mike had off. The two of us began clocking out at work, clocking in at home, on opposite schedules.

I hid in the world of my lighthouse novel. Tucked myself inside the body of Anna, my main character, one paragraph at a time in the dark cornered aerospace lab until I wasn't there anymore. I was bent over a shitty Evinrude that crapped out in the middle of the channel as a storm whipped up. I was slowly solving the mystery, realizing William Harris was Kyle's dad. I was dropping trees for firewood, smoking a hundred pounds of salmon and canning it for the winter. I was free.

YEAR EIGHT

CHAPTER FOURTEEN

Mike was at the firehouse the first night I tried the eighth or ninth new drug. A couple hours after swallowing the first dose, I bolted upright to the sound of a strangled cry. Nate had reactive airway disease, and I knew before my feet hit the ground that he was having trouble breathing. "I'm coming, buddy," I called as the room spun and swayed, and I pulled my way, hand over hand, through it: along the dresser, the wall, the doorframe.

In his room, I untangled him from Wes and took him out into the living room to figure out if the drugs we had on hand could help or if he needed a mad dash to the ER. He gagged, so I moved us to the kitchen sink. I reached for the light switch, holding him as he puked in the sink. When the room flooded with light, I could see the scary way the base of his throat constricted as he struggled to pull in air. This was the sign we needed to get to the hospital as quickly as possible. I pulled him against my chest and turned back toward the bedroom to grab his brother.

The wood floor came out of nowhere. My head bounced, and I fought against the dark edges of my vision closing in. "No," I heard myself say from far away. There had been several previous rushes to the hospital, and when he was this bad, he didn't have long. My vision pinpricked and then blacked out.

I woke up on the floor with Nate clinging to my chest. His pale skin had tinged blue, and he was convulsing now in his effort to get in enough air. My vision was still dark at the edges, so I kept my head low, scrambled to my feet, grabbed his brother, and ran to the car, bent over in bare feet. I strapped the one chest strap each, peeled out of the driveway, and ran a red light.

In front of the ER, I left the car running, unbuckled Nate, and ran through the sliding glass door. The front desk person met me just inside the doors, and soon, there were doctors and nurses everywhere and someone was taking him from me and I was reaching for the nearest wall to right the room.

"Mama?" Wes had gotten himself out of the car, his nighttime diaper wet and hanging thick in his jammies that were tight across his round little belly. His favorite stuffed giraffe hung by one foot from his tiny hand. "Where's NayNay?" The car doors hung open behind him, the car parked at a haphazard angle. He was on the verge of tears.

I scooped Wes up, held him tight against my chest. "He's okay now, buddy. The doctors are helping." The room uncertain, I kept a shoulder to the wall and moved toward the double doors the doctors and nurses had disappeared behind with Nate, the tether between the three of us stretching uncomfortably across the distance. I breathed in the grounding smell of the skin in the crook of Wes's neck, focused on his heartbeat against mine as we moved toward the room where Nate had already been hooked up to a breathing mask, someone jabbing a needle into his chubby thigh, both Wes and I reaching for him.

CHAPTER FIFTEEN

I sent the novel off to Susan and avoided my inbox until I couldn't stand it anymore and then checked it obsessively every hour.

Three weeks after I'd sent it off, an email showed up from her with nothing in the subject line. It was 10:00 p.m., and I was in the lab testing the descent brake that would go up with the next Mars rover and hopefully keep it from crashing to the surface of Mars when it was deployed.

There had been a number of issues in the engineering of it, we were behind schedule for the launch, and everyone was nervous. The testing needed to go without a hitch, I needed to keep the chamber within the exact parameters of temperature within 0.1 degrees or this very expensive experiment would be chalked up to one big failure of the company. The lead engineer hovered at the edges of the lab as I ran the chambers.

I stared at my inbox. Wouldn't she have put something encouraging in the subject line if the email was good? It was midnight in New York. Perhaps she'd put off telling me the book still was a mess until the last thing because she felt sorry for me. I started at it for another twenty minutes and then clicked it open.

In big, bold letters, she wrote, "You did it!!!! Call me tomorrow."

"AHHHH!!!!" I screamed. I'm not a screamer. "HOLY SHIT!!!!"

The engineer came running around the corner. "What? What is it? What happened?"

I was half standing over my computer, still staring at the words, making sure I hadn't imagined them. "I did it!!"

"Did what? Did something happen?"

I peeled my eyes away from my email to look at him. His face was a wreck. He looked like he was holding his breath. "My book!" I told him. "This is an even bigger deal than going to Mars!" I grabbed my phone and ran outside to call Mike.

The next day on the phone, Susan said, "I can't believe how much work you put into this draft. It's incredible. Brilliant to make William Harris Kyle's dad."

"Oh. Ah," I wanted to come clean about all of it—the dizziness, the babies—but figured I'd start here. I scrunched up my nose and admitted, "Mike came up with it."

She laughed. "Does he write also?"

"No. He drinks beer. Does this mean his name has to go on the front cover along with mine?"

■ ■ ■

A year into the every-three-month drug trials, Susan called.

"Ig Publishing wants to buy your book. I think we should go with their offer."

I'd just pulled up in front of the house. The boys were in their car seats behind me, asleep in the hot, sweaty way of car naps.

I slipped out of the car so as not to wake them. Both sleeping at the same time was always a small miracle. Under the bright Colorado sun, I squealed into the phone, "Yes, oh my god, yes, whatever the offer is, yes."

Susan laughed. "So you're sure? You want to hear more?"

"Yes. No. I have to call Mike."

She got in a few short sentences before I got her off the phone.

"Mike!" I yelled when he picked up. I was pacing in the street now.

"Are you okay?" he asked. "The kids?"

"Fine, they're fine. Susan sold my book. For . . . well, we're not rich. Sorry."

Mike whooped and hollered and got on the firehouse PA system. "Rach sold her book!!!" In the background, the crew cheered.

■ ■ ■

Eighteen months into the every-three-month drug trials, Susan called again.

"Just got off the phone with Robert. He heard from *Oprah Magazine*."

I was sitting on the edge of the tub with a bag of peanut M&M's as bribes for both boys, who had been sitting on their plastic potties in front of me for at least forty-five minutes doing everything except going pee or poo.

"Oprah?" I froze, a green M&M halfway to my mouth.

"They picked *Point of Direction* for their list of top ten books to pick up now."

"What?" There was only 10 percent of my brain left functional between the dizziness that day and trying to get at least one of my toddlers to get the hang of wearing underwear. Surely, I'd heard wrong.

"Congrats!" Susan said.

"Wait. For reals?"

Suan laughed. "Yes!" I let out a whoop way too loud for the small bathroom, and the boys clapped and cheered from their potties.

■ ■ ■

The lighthouse book, with its new fancy title, *Point of Direction,* was scheduled for release in May 2014. In April 2014, the American Booksellers Association picked it as a top ten debut. Susan called to say I was to fly out to be a part of their annual conference in just a few weeks.

The dizziness does not like air travel, talking to people I don't know, big crowds, noisy rooms, conference room lighting, elevators, or long days. I threw a couple shirts in a suitcase and hoped for the best. I boarded a 737, but it might as well have been a bush plane. I was headed for Seattle, but I might as well have stepped off the plane into the backcountry of Alaska without a radio. I expected at any moment for the dizziness to attack like a bear, flatten me like a falling tree, or swallow me whole like a shadowy crevasse.

I kept my eyes as still as possible the whole plane ride, found the service stairs to get to my room on the twenty-third floor and back down again for the evening book signing, said no thanks to the glass of wine, and still I was dizzier than ever. The packed, high ceilinged conference room rolled and sloshed and slid uncontrollably. I glanced around, located the nearest trash cans in case I puked. A very nice woman introduced herself and explained she was taking authors to their tables. I followed her to a table in a long row of black tableclothed author tables. But this one had stacks of my book piled up on top of it.

"That's my book," I breathed out.

She glanced at me. "Sure is," she said. The conference was for independent booksellers who came together to check out the year's new releases to help them decide what to stock in their bookstores.

"I haven't seen it yet," I said, picking up the top book in the closest stack. On the cover was the actual lighthouse the ferry went past that day years before I had ever been dizzy. The picture is foggy and moody and perfect. I held in my hands an actual printed book with my name on the cover. I pressed it to my chest. How had I done this? I could hardly breathe. I'd done it. Despite the all day everyday, hateful dizziness, I wanted to drop to my knees, cry for how hard I had worked, for all the times I had wanted to give up but didn't. For how unlikely it was to be standing here.

"You'll just need to sit down here," the poor woman who was in charge of me said, possibly more than a little weirded out that I was still hugging my book like a life raft. The conference room was packed with other authors sitting at their tables in front of their books, long lines forming of booksellers who wanted a free signed copy.

Still white-knuckling the book in one hand, I used the other to navigate around the edge of the table without toppling over and sat down like some sort of wide eyed alien just arrived on Earth.

The author to my left held in her hand the type of pen you might get as a graduation gift and was smiling and chatting up the guy in the tweed jacket who seemed truly thrilled to be getting a copy of her book.

I dug around in my bag to see if I had a pen. I found one I'd stolen from the bank. But that was okay, no one was coming over to get a book anyway. I peeled the book from where it was still pressed tightly to my chest and stared at my name on the cover.

"Rachel?" I was making the woman in charge of me nervous.

"Sorry," I said, accepting the book she was handing me from the stack, accurately reading the situation to determine I was not parting with the one I had in my clutches. She opened the book in her hands to the cover page. There was suddenly a line forming. The guy in the front said, "I own the bookstore in Palmer, Alaska. I'm really excited about this one. Jim Kennedy," he prompted, pointing at where I was supposed to sign his copy.

I looked down at the page. The only thing that was coming to me were things you'd write in a yearbook.

Love ya like a sister!

Have a great summer!

I breathed out. Tried to make room for something else to pop up in my head. *Dear Jim,* I scribbled through the crushing noise in the room, the fog in my head, through the swaying chair underneath me, none of which mattered at all.

■ ■ ■

Two years into the every-three-month drug trials, I woke up feeling like someone had my heart in a vise. Mike was at work, so I struggled through the breakfast making, the every other minute disputes between the boys. I wasn't supposed to have a heart attack until I was forty-five but was not at all surprised that it was early. I wondered if Dad had this heart in a vise feeling the day of the softball game.

I loaded up the boys and we drove to the firehouse. They loved to visit Da-Da, to put on the headsets and pretend to drive the fire truck.

"Hey, little mans!" Mike bent down just inside the bay door, and they ran into his arms on chubby legs when we got to the firehouse. Both started talking at him at once, telling him all sorts of important bits of info he'd missed while he was at work the previous day. The boys began to chase each other around the fire truck, another favorite firehouse activity.

"You alright?" he asked, pulling me into a hug.

I shook my head. "My heart," I said. "Feels like someone is squeezing it." I was leaning over a bit to accommodate it.

"Jesus. Why didn't you go to the ER?" He shuffled me into the back of the ambulance.

"What was I going to do with the boys at the ER?"

He hooked me up to the EKG. Six small wires attached to my chest with big, round sticky pads. The boys continued to lap the firetruck, squealing and laughing while we sat in the small, cramped space of the ambulance. I studied his face as he studied the valleys and peaks on the small screen. *I'm sorry*, I wanted to whisper. *I'm so sorry I am happening to you.*

He squinted at the screen, turned a knob, and pushed at buttons. I listened to my children laugh, watched the worry gather at the edges of Mike's eyes, thought about my dad dead in the dirt.

"It's fine," he finally said with relief, sitting back. "It's fine. But you have to make an appointment with a GP today to get checked out."

Both boys broke into screams of pain when they crashed into each other. Mike pulled me into a tight hug. There was so much to say and no way to say it. We quickly pulled the tape from my chest and climbed out of the ambulance to attend to the boys, who had bonked heads and had matching angry red bumps. They both screamed and clutched their heads and writhed around, and I wished I could do the exact same thing.

The following day, a GP hooked me up to a much larger, fancier EKG. I sat on the edge of the exam table, the crinkly paper sticking to my hands where I held on tight, afraid I might fall off with the way the room slipped and slid around me. It was a relief almost to be in a doctor's office and not have to present some vague, floaty symptom.

"All looks normal," she said. She unhooked me from the EKG and stood in front of me, head tilted. "The type of chest pain you are having is caused by stress."

She pressed her lips together and smashed up her eyebrows. "This is your body telling you it's time to make some significant changes."

■ ■ ■

A couple weeks later, at my next appointment with the marathon runner migraine doctor, I told her about the heart vise, which had not gone away. My body had taken to curling itself around my heart so that I no longer stood or sat up straight. From my hunched over position on the chair, I flung my hand at the list of drugs, more than half of them starred, notes scribbled in the margins. "Do I have vestibular migraine or not?"

Weirdly, she was sitting on the paper covered exam table. Her feet didn't reach the ground, and she had a hand on either side of each knee, her arms straight, leaned forward a bit as if she were about to launch. She could probably tell I wasn't going to make it from the chair to the exam table.

"You don't have migraine," she said. "I'm not even convinced vestibular migraine is a thing."

"Then how do you explain why so many migraine drugs take the edge off the dizziness?" It was so cold in the prison cell, and I was so alone.

The doctor breathed out a heavy breath. "All the drugs we use for migraine are designed for different things. There's no drug designed specifically for migraine. Maybe you have other issues that those drugs were addressing, but you don't have migraine."

"Then what do I have?"

"I have no idea." She paused for a minute, sorry, I could tell, in the way of someone who'd never lost control.

Once, at work in Alaska, I was hiking up an abandoned Forest Service road on an uninhabited island. It was raining sideways and the wind was kicked up. Just before I got to the top of a hill, a deer appeared at the crest of the hill, running straight for me. Her tongue hung out too far, her eyes were open too much, and her legs seemed unsteady, her knees bending in odd ways. Despite all this, she was hurtling herself up and over the hill at top speed. I rolled into a ditch to keep from getting trampled. As I got to my knees in the tall grasses, a wolf topped the hill a few feet away. The wolf's eyes slid over to me. He was thin and rangy, needed the meat. He locked his eyes back on the deer and trotted past, barely breathing hard, letting the deer run, staying far enough back that perhaps she had the thought that she might just make it. That she might just get back to wherever her young were bedded down.

When the wolf disappeared around the bend at the bottom of the hill, I got back to my feet. A few minutes later, the final shriek of the deer filled the forest.

■ ■ ■

I needed a GP to help me figure out where to turn next. I was out of ideas. I read through the bios of the other docs at the family practice clinic where I'd gotten the EKG. I skipped over where they went to school and read the last paragraph, where they invariably said something like, "loves to mountain bike and scrapbook in her free time." I found nothing useful, so I picked based on who looked the nicest in their picture.

I tried to relax as I waited in the overly lit room. I was the only one who could hear the wolf behind me.

The doctor came in, all smiles and friendly hellos, just as nice as she looked in her picture. She sat across from me on the rolly chair, listened carefully, and read the whole spreadsheet. She folded in on herself a bit as she read, poring over all the diagnoses to date. As she read, I stared out the window at the parking lot. Tried hard not to place too much hope in her. If she could just divert the wolf's attention, give me just a bit more breathing room.

The doctor set the spreadsheet down and sighed. "If thirty-three other doctors haven't been able to figure this out, I'm not going to be able to either."

■ ■ ■

One week later, I was in a hotel room in the mountains with two writer friends. They sat in chairs. I lay on the bed. They were only sort-of friends. To have actual friends, you have to be able to do things. Go out, hold conversations. I wanted them both to be actual friends, but that was beyond my reach.

The three of us were teaching at a weekend writing conference. The two-hour class I had just finished teaching had taken everything out of me. To push through the dizziness for that long, to pretend to be fine, to think through the mind fog enough to make sense to a room full of students had left me strung out, like I'd been hiking through the night, lost, at the height of bear season.

One of the women was talking about her medical struggles with early onset MS. I listened, sunk in a bed of seasick misery. I wanted to participate in the conversation, to commune about what it was like to struggle through days. I missed hanging out with friends, feeling any sort of shared experience with anyone. With my eyes closed, the room spun faster, formed a vortex with a bottomless hole that everything was disappearing into. Their conversation stretched so far from me I couldn't reach it.

The woman with MS said, "I had to come home early. I couldn't handle another day of it." A canceled book tour for her recently released memoir. "It was too hard. All my symptoms flared, and I had to get back home where I could rest."

"I feel like that every day." I couldn't meet their eyes. "Except there's nowhere to go that would be better. I'm 100 percent useless. My children and husband would be better off without me." I'd turned into a geyser gushing gross, awkward stuff after years of dormancy.

The air in the room turned brittle. The gross, gushy stuff dripped down the walls.

"You don't mean it," the one without MS said.

But I did. Definitively, for the first time.

YEAR NINE

CHAPTER SIXTEEN

A few nights later, on my way home from the lab at midnight, I stopped at the railroad tracks. The moon was out, and the cows hulked in the cold field off to my left. The tracks stretched into the distance, the train somewhere else. I touched my forehead to the frosted over glass of the side window, thought about the soft pudge of Wes's forearm, Nate's big belly laugh that got us all laughing, Mike's body against mine in the early morning hours.

I dropped my hand to the latch to open the door, held it there. The train would be on schedule as it always was, set to pound past this particular intersection in eight minutes.

The fact that multiple migraine drugs had affected the dizziness had to mean something. I watched the moonlight glint off the tracks.

In one final, knock kneed push up and over the top of the hill, I returned my hands to the steering wheel. I would try one more migraine doctor to see if he/she/they agreed it wasn't vestibular migraine.

And then I would let myself be done.

■ ■ ■

The next morning, I put a movie on for the boys and sat down at the computer. I would have to be quick. Too much screen time would kick the dizziness into a storm that I couldn't parent through.

I made a few decisions first. I wasn't driving to Denver, and I wasn't going to put myself through the agony of reading the website text about the doctor or the clinic. Every one of them said the same shit about being patient centered, as if they all hired the same copy editor anyway.

Three migraine clinics came up within a ten-mile radius of my house. I closed my eyes to let the added amount of dizziness settle and then clicked through the pictures of the providers at each clinic. I picked the guy who looked the least like a jackass.

I dialed the clinic's number. As the phone rang, I told myself I could endure three more months while I waited for this appointment. A decision settled over me like a weighted blanket, with the sounds of Pooh and Tigger in the background: If he tells me I do not have vestibular migraine, as the marathon runner has posited, and returns me to the hellscape of no diagnosis, I won't see any more doctors. If he tells me I do have vestibular migraine and repeats what Vandy said about Verapamil being the only option, I won't see any more doctors. I'll let the wolf catch me.

"Can you come in this Thursday?" the woman who answered the phone asked.

"What?" No one ever had an appointment that soon. Probably because he was the worst doctor ever and no one ever went back. But I was too tired to step back into the spinning world wide web and pick a different doctor.

"Okay," I said.

■ ■ ■

His office was on the same horseshoe road as the painfully young chiropractor with the cold metal roller. I sat in the waiting room and stared at the *People* magazine. Jennifer Aniston and her relationship problems jumped and jerked on the cover. I followed a medical assistant to a small room and waited some more with my eyes closed. This is the last time, I kept telling myself, trying to feel the relief of it. I didn't even bother bringing the spreadsheet.

The doctor had on jeans and an untucked polo shirt and shoes he probably wore on the weekends. He sat down on the rolly thing and looked at me. I hit the highlights in one long run-on sentence and finished up with, "I just need to know if you think it's migraine or if you agree with the last migraine doctor that it's not." A cold fear spread in my chest. This was it.

"Alright," he said, slow and easy. The overhead florescent lights were turned off, and the shades were drawn tight. The room was lit with soft lamps in the corners. The far edges of me became a little less jagged as I relaxed into the calm space of the room.

The doctor skipped over what my grandmother died of and instead asked me about the quality of my sleep, the exact dimensions of the dizziness. The computer sat untouched, the doctor leaned back against the wall, folded his hands, as if we had all the time in the world to get to know each other, to untangle the tangled mess before us. When I came to the end of the answer to one of his questions, he waited, allowing me the time my brain needed to land on the right words, to sort through what I was trying to say.

In addition to what drugs the previous migraine doctor had tried and what happened with each, he asked if I was able to eat, to parent, to read.

"I think you have vestibular migraine," he said after an hour in that gently lit room, still watching me closely.

My vision began to tunnel. The room loosened and began to swing and sway wildly.

He went on. "I'd like to give you two shots that we use to treat vestibular migraine all the time."

All the time? As in, there were a lot of people with this problem? No one had mentioned shots before.

"So you think vestibular migraine is a thing?"

He laughed. "Yes. I think vestibular migraine is a thing. We could give the shots a try right now," he said. He made no move for the door. Still looked relaxed leaned up against the wall. He waited for me to agree or disagree. "See what happens," he added.

I knew what was going to happen. The dizziness would get worse. A shot wasn't a drug you could stop taking the next day if you got some horrendous side effect. A shot could last days or weeks. "I don't have a ride home if I can't drive," I said. Mike was at work. "I only have a babysitter for two hours."

He watched me. Not in a calculating, mind-whirring, get-it-done-and-move-on-to-the-next-patient kind of way, but in a looks-like-this-sucks-for-you kind of way. "I think the combination of the two drugs will help you. And if for some reason it makes you worse, we'll make sure you get home."

Fear pounded through me. I knew for sure I could not handle feeling any worse than I already did. That my ability to meet the needs of my kids was hanging on by a thread. That I was hanging on by a thread.

The doctor was still watching me, but I'd run out of the ability to articulate. But it didn't matter. He seemed to read it in my slumped shoulders, the grip I had on the chair, in whatever my face was doing. "I think we should start with these two shots and see if you respond. I honestly think you will." He sat there, holding some of the weight of the dizziness long enough that I could get a deep breath, make a clear decision.

I nodded my assent and decided I'd sleep off the effects in my car until I was safe to drive home. I would text the babysitter and ask if she could stay longer.

"Great," he said. "And then I'd like to see you twice a week for the foreseeable future. Lots to sort out here."

I stared at him, dumbfounded. Here was the first offer to address what was happening on the surface and to hold the space for all that was going on underneath it. To keep close tabs on the whereabouts of my body and my brain. Twice a week sorting was a recognition of how bad it was, how desperately I needed the support not only as a patient but as a person.

The doctor left the room, and the medical assistant returned and administered the injections. Sumatriptan and Toradol, she explained. I paid the copay, made it down the stairs, and sat in my car in my winter coat with both windows down. I could have stayed in the exam room, but the mix of hope and terror was too much. I needed to breathe outside air.

Within five minutes, the brick wall of the doctor's two-story office building stilled. The constant dull throb of my head lessened. The heavy fog in my mind broke up like ice in spring. I looked at the steering wheel. It was still. I got out of the car, stared at the sidewalk, the bare branches of the trees. Everything was still. I spread my hand out in front of me and stared at it. I took a tentative step. The ground was solid. I dared to watch a car drive by on the horseshoe street. Tracking the motion did not cause me to slosh or spin. I watched another car just to be sure. No spinning. No sloshing. I walked to the middle of the parking lot and stared up at the trees, the sky, all of it new and fucking glorious.

I should cry, I thought. *I should drop to my knees like a shipwrecked person returned to land.*

Terrified suddenly that it wouldn't last, I rushed back to my car. I needed to get home, to hug my children, be present with them for the first time ever, drive down to the firehouse and sit as close as possible to Mike.

■ ■ ■

It didn't last for long, but it didn't matter. It lasted long enough for hope to turn into something big and solid. Something more substantial than a balloon.

I continued to see Dr. Tanner twice a week as he worked to smooth out the huge knot my nervous system had worked its way into. It didn't happen fast.

In the two years I spent at the migraine clinic with the vacuum sealed doctor, she spent thirty minutes at the intake appointment and then ten minutes every three months after that. Which means, in two years, we spent just over an hour and a half together.

In the first week of my care, Dr. Tanner and I spent two hours together. He asked question after question, like a detective on the path of a hardened criminal.

Each week, he stretched and pulled at my back and neck to relieve the tension stored there. He adjusted my neck according to his osteopathic training and continually adjusted the combinations of my meds. Some helped, some didn't. I continued to suffer all the side effects. As he calmed things down with a delicate combination of pharmaceuticals, the physical adjustments began to work.

I was still at the bottom of a deep dark hole, but he'd opened the hatch door at the top. I could see the light, the staircase leading up. I took one slow step at a time, fell back down a bunch, but always, he was there at the top, relaxed in his weekend shoes, keeping a close eye on my progress.

He explained that migraine doesn't have to be a headache and aura. It can present as dizziness. That sound and light sensitivity are part of it. That elevated histamines would further agitate an already overwhelmed nervous system. When I reported back that whatever drug we tried wasn't working, he shook it off quickly, didn't force a three-month trial, asked a bunch more questions, set our sights on another possible solution.

We talked and schemed and worked at the knot, meeting twice a week in that middle ground between sick and healthy. It's not easy for either patient or doctor to get to that middle ground, or for either party to stay there for any length of time. It's hard to sit with someone else's misery for an hour, and it's horrible to make yourself so vulnerable that another person can see all the angles from which you suffer. It's hard to know what to advise for a person obviously so fragile and twisted up, and it's hard to trust the advice when it might wreck you for months.

I still had bad days, but I no longer had bad weeks, bad years. I was still fragile—easily knocked down a stair or two by weather systems, by a bad night's sleep, by a birthday party full of happily screaming kids.

The depression was still there, gathering like a rainstorm sometimes, but not all the time.

Whole days passed in which I was consumed by how lovely it is to grocery shop without nausea, how nice it is to drive at night with the windows down past fields of still horses, how wonderful to tip my head back in laughter without causing the room to spin.

I delighted in the ability to curl up with my boys and read them a bedtime story. In the relief that settled on Mike's face. In how much easier parenting is when you don't feel terrible.

YEAR TEN

CHAPTER SEVENTEEN

The dizziness did not loosen its grip easily. It got violent. A couple of times, it knocked me almost back to the bottom of the staircase. Each time this happened, Dr. Tanner would sigh, pull up a chair, and sit with my black mood, patiently untangling what he'd untangled before. Asking me questions, reading the subtext like a person trying to follow a messed up plot in a novel, handing me a box of tissues, once, when I was certain I was hiding the fact that I felt like crying.

In the midst of one of those chest shoves to the bottom of the staircase, I sat outside on our deck, trying to convince myself that this would pass, that Dr. Tanner would not give up on me, that I would not be stuck at the bottom forever. I heard little feet racing through the kitchen. In the way of five-year-olds, Wes was convinced he knew sign language. He would move his hands and arms around in elaborate gestures that sometimes involved his hips and then quiz me on what he'd just said. Usually it was, "Can I have some milk?" or, "I love Mama."

On that particularly bad dizzy day, he came racing out onto the back deck with the look on his face that meant *here comes some sign language!* I took a deep breath and tried to focus on him through the fog. My head hurt bad enough that the ache had moved into my teeth. Fear stomped around, pounding my insides flat as I rode the endless roller coaster of illness.

I opened my arms, and Wes ran into them and then bounced back and stood in front of me. I left one hand on either of his hips, wanting more than anything to protect him from the way life can rob you of yourself with no forewarning, wanting more than anything to be a mom who could backpack, who could take him skiing. I smiled and stuffed it all deep down where I hoped he couldn't feel the weight of it.

"Hi, buddy."

He wriggled out of my loose embrace, jostling from foot to foot. He rubbed away his wild-eyed smile with his little hands and settled into a serious face. Sign language, as always, was a serious matter.

I resisted the urge to reach out and touch him again. He felt so far away, the vast, dark, swirling matter of dizziness stretching between us. *I will not lose him to this*, I told myself for the thousandth time and began the process of clawing my way toward him.

He started with a palms up, wide armed gesture, his chin jutted out, that in the adult world usually means "What the fuck?"

But he'd decided a while back that this particular move meant "Mama."

"Mama," I said, decoding.

"Yes!" he screeched and danced around in the red and yellow leaves accumulated on the deck. He raced back to his position in front of me, dropped his face back into the serious look. Next, he held out one hand, palm down, put all the fingers of his other hand underneath, and turned them in a slow circle. This was a new one.

"What's that the sign for?" I asked.

He dropped his hands and pulled his face into a slow smile, his white blonde hair a wild map of how he'd slept the night before. The deck snaked like a river underneath him. I closed one eye, wondered how much longer I could keep up the facade for him.

He peered into my eyes and said, "That means, I will love you when you're all twisted up."

YEAR ELEVEN

CHAPTER EIGHTEEN

A letter from the insurance company arrived to let me know my current medical care was under review. This was nothing new. Turns out when you start using your insurance, they start reviewing everything. They start claiming that someone removing a chunk of earwax is surgery, that checking your cholesterol is an experimental procedure, and deny coverage.

A sinking feeling piled up on top of the dizziness that they'd quit paying for Dr. Tanner, but how could they argue with this one? I was no longer undergoing expensive tests that they had to pay for, it was just me and Dr. Tanner sitting in a dimly lit room twice a week, trying to figure things out. I recycled the letter.

■ ■ ■

Six months later, while I was sitting in the waiting room at Dr. Tanner's, the office manager, Louise, called me into her office. She is kind and calm, the sort of person you might call in an emergency. She lowered herself into her chair behind her tidy desk, and I cautiously perched on a chair in the tight space next to the door. The look on her face made my throat clog.

"Your insurance company has decided your care here is not medically necessary." She drummed her fingers against the desk.

"Okay," I said, trying to clear my throat. "Clearly, it is medically necessary."

"Clearly," she agreed. "It's going into a second review. They've asked for all your medical records, and I'm going to need you to write up something in which you explain that the care you get from Dr. Tanner is, in your view, medically necessary."

I wrote a two-page letter in which I explained the number of doctors, the fact that seven minutes every three months got me nowhere, the years of hopelessness and depression that wore me paper thin. I wrote about all the things I could do that I had not been able to do for a decade: drive with two eyes open, run multiple errands in a row, read for over half a day, and tolerate a computer for an hour or two. I wrote that while all of this was glorious, I was nowhere near healthy and that without Dr. Tanner, all of it would slip away. I mentioned how close the railroad tracks were. I included my spreadsheet.

■ ■ ■

Six months later, Louise called me in again. I sank into the small chair in the narrow space next to the door. This time, my throat clogged up, and the dizziness loosened the walls before Louise even spoke. She pinched her lips together and then said, "An expert in the field reviewed your records and determined the care you get here is not medically necessary. It's going into a third review. I'm going to need more than a letter from you for this one. Here's a letter your insurance company sent with everything we have to send in and the dates everything is due by. The highlighted ones are what I need you to gather up." She handed over a single sheet, and my eyes locked on a line at the top: "Outstanding Balance = $75,000."

"Wait," I said through the pounding of my heart. "This is what I owe the insurance company?"

"No," Louise said with a toss of her hand. "No. That's what your insurance company owes us."

"They haven't been paying you?"

"Not . . . for a while now," she said. "But it's nothing to worry over," she added quickly.

My ears began to ring. "So I owe you $75,000?" Mike and I would have to get divorced. While I had about two hundred dollars to my name, he had a retirement account with lots of zeros. We'd get divorced, I would be slapped with the medical bill, declare bankruptcy, and be financially ruined while his hard earned money remained his. And maybe it was better if we were divorced anyway. He could be free of the never ending illness roller coaster. I would move into a dump of an apartment full of roaches, and he could keep the kids safe and fed.

"No," Louise said interrupting the spool of my mind. "Dr. Tanner is not going to hold you responsible for that. And besides, insurance companies do this and then cave in at the last minute and pay it off, or at least some portion of it. Don't worry, we'll file the review and it'll work out."

I walked back out into the waiting room in a haze. Nothing to do with the dizziness typically "worked out." My whole body buzzed with anxiety as I was led back to the exam room to wait for Dr. Tanner. As soon as he walked in, I said, "I don't have $75,000."

He laughed, his eyes crinkling up in the corners. "Who does?" He'd joined the army out of high school, had lived in a tent for some part of medical school.

"I'm serious," I said. He closed the door and sat down on the rolly chair. "I didn't know my insurance company hasn't been paying you for a whole year." I felt like a snake in the grass who'd just been exposed.

Dr. Tanner shrugged one shoulder.

"I can't keep coming here, racking up more unpaid visits."

He looked up. We both knew where that would likely lead.

"I'll start paying out of pocket. What do you charge?"

Dr. Tanner shook his head. After twice a week chats over two years, he likely could guess at my financial situation. He knew Mike was a fireman, that I hadn't gone to law school or done anything else that would have garnered the ability to pay out of pocket for twice a week doctor's appointments.

He tilted his head slightly, still shaking it. "We'll just keep fighting it. We'll get them to pay some portion of it at least. Louise says there's still a third review to go through."

Relief flooded me, but I felt snaky still. "It could be a hundred thousand dollars by the time they finish up a third review."

He smiled. "They'll likely pay it. And if not, they'll settle, and we'll get something. Don't worry about it."

But I did worry about it. Late at night especially. Each morning, I woke with lead in my veins at the idea that I might soon get cut off from the one person who might possibly see me through to a life worth living. I started to think up moneymaking schemes to pay for my medical care. I would deliver pizzas. I would write a romance novel. Except that up to that point in my writing, I'd avoided sex scenes like the plague.

I looked up how much buying my own insurance would cost. Triple what we currently paid through Mike's job and way more than we had. I would get a job somewhere that offered me insurance. I would be some asshole's secretary. Fine. Except, how was I going to hide that looking at a computer screen all day long wasn't a possibility? Neither were spreadsheets, Google searches, or walking on patterned carpet. And I didn't own a skirt. Or nice shoes.

I made phone calls, guffawed at how much each doctor's office charged to print my medical records, and tried hard not to call each receptionist a rat bastard. I made myself exorbitantly dizzy researching and printing off peer reviewed research that showed every single drug and the osteopathic work Dr. Tanner used to treat me were all standard care, all FDA approved, all viable treatments for severe chronic migraine.

I wrote a longer letter to describe in more detail what I'd been through, how much I had improved since being treated by Dr. Tanner.

I requested all the documentation from the first two reviews the insurance company had conducted, which arrived in a two-foot-by-two-foot box filled to the rim. I pored over the two previous review letters by the insurance company that determined my care medically unnecessary and rebutted each point with cited data. I studied their stated review procedure and looked for any ways in which they hadn't followed it.

I discovered that my insurance company—who I really want to name here but won't; I will say it's one of the big ones and that a bunch of you are covered by them too—anyway, they own a company, which we'll call X, who hires medical professionals to review patient medical records and determine whether or not their current care (which is typically flagged because it's costing the insurance company a pretty penny) is medically necessary. The insurance company, through X company, which they own, pays these medical professionals to say whether or not the patient's care is necessary.

Now, if you are a medical professional who keeps telling the insurance company, *Yes, this person's care is necessary, and so is this other person's and this other person's*, it stands to reason that the insurance company would no longer employ you to review records. It stands to reason that if you were someone who continually said, *No, this is not medically necessary, therefore, you should stop paying for this person's care*, your sweet side gig stays intact and you keep raking in the extra cash each month.

The medical professional hired to review my case as part of the second review was a nameless nurse. Not a nurse practitioner. Not a nurse who had worked in a migraine clinic for twenty-five years. Just a nurse. Which you can become with a two-year degree. Maybe she was brilliant, or maybe she just needed the extra cash for her kid's summer camp. She determined that my care from Dr. Tanner was not medically necessary. What a surprise.

In their procedurals, the insurance company says if they deem a third review necessary, they will, this time, hire a professional in the field of diagnosis to review the medical records to determine the necessity of treatment or not. That medical professional will remain confidential. Except, in that giant box of papers was the signed report by the doctor who determined my care from Dr. Tanner was medically unnecessary.

It wasn't just that this doctor was yanking Dr. Tanner from my life. It stood to reason that if our insurance wouldn't pay for the FDA approved drugs and treatments administered in Dr. Tanner's office, they wouldn't cover them if they were administered by any other doctor's office either. They were essentially saying, *We don't care that it took you a decade to land on what works, you can't have it anymore. From anyone. Even though you pay your monthly premiums. You do your part, but don't expect us to do ours.*

I stared at the name. How could a doctor, in good faith, make major medical decisions for me without ever talking to me? I googled him. Found his phone number.

A bright receptionist answered in his office in Pittsburgh.

"Hi," I said. "I've just moved to the Pittsburgh area and I'd like to establish care with a new migraine doctor. Does Dr. Z (I really, really, really want to write his name here) see patients with vestibular migraine?"

"Vestibular migraine?" she said, as if I'd asked if he treated martians. "No. I mean, every once in a while, he'll treat patients with migraine, but I've never heard of vestibular migraine. This is a chronic pain clinic. I think you'd be better off under the care of someone else."

■ ■ ■

Six months later, I had progressed to seeing Dr. Tanner once a week. I was moving in the right direction again. Still underground but steadily climbing stairs. I was still dizzy every day, but it didn't rage out of control as often. But there was still a long way to go.

On a bright spring morning, I got home after having walked the boys to their elementary school, and Mike was sitting at the kitchen table with an unopened letter from my insurance company that was undoubtedly their final decision about whether or not my current plan of care was medically necessary. Mike looked blown out, tired from running calls through the previous two nights. He'd gotten off shift that morning at 7:00 a.m. and collected the mail on his way in.

My hands began to shake. "I can't open it," I said. How would we afford individual insurance for me? We both drove old cars, we both worked, we lived in a small house, our boys weren't signed up for expensive camps or day care. We lived within our means, and still, paying for insurance on the open market wasn't attainable.

I felt trapped, wild. I wanted to buy a ticket to Pittsburgh and shove a picture of my kids in the face of the doctor who'd checked the box that read "medically unnecessary" and collected his $1,500 or whatever. *These kids will suffer the consequence of your action*, I wanted to tell him.

"It'll be fine," Mike said, his eyes deeply creased. "Whatever it says," he picked up my hand. "We'll just deal with it. Together. Okay?"

I watched him for a minute. I'd tried so hard to keep this problem my problem so that he wouldn't run, but he never would've run. I stepped into his arms. He pulled me in tight, and something in me broke. For the first time since that humid night in front of the hospital when I was seventeen years old, I let myself trust in that other side of the probability. That I could love someone, need them, and they would come home from the softball game.

Still leaned up against Mike, I opened the letter slowly. It stated succinctly that our insurance company would no longer pay for care from Dr. Tanner. They would let me go once every three months for Botox, which we'd recently discovered helped, but if I went to see him for any other reason, I was on my own to pay for that. No more weekly shots that helped me more than anything else that can't be administered at home, no more follow-up appointments to adjust meds. I would, however, still be expected to pay my monthly premium.

I spent the rest of the day in a dizzy, anxiety-ridden haze. In and out of bed, not eating, watching the walls slide up in my vision, followed by the floor. I needed a full-time job with no screens that would give me health insurance. The post office, I decided. But I'd have to find out which health insurance company they use. And what if they changed every year in January like the aerospace company did? I would have to take the chance that they wouldn't switch to my current insurance company, and if they did, I'd have to quit and get a different job.

Until then, I could sort mail in the big open warehouse part of the post office, work my way up to my own route. Maybe a walking one so that I could be outside all day. I could do that. I would be alright. Mike would not go broke because of me. The kids would have to go to after school care on the days Mike worked. It wouldn't be the end of the world. I went to after school care. It was like *Lord of the Flies*, but so is the rest of the world.

I looked up how to apply for a job at the post office, but the dizziness was raging with such ferocity, the screen kept slipping to the left, and I couldn't get the cursor where I needed it to be. I gave up and called Louise to ask if I could meet with both her and Dr. Tanner that afternoon.

■ ■ ■

We all three squeezed into Louise's office. Dr. Tanner stood up against the wall, his hands tucked behind his back. It took everything I had to talk without sputter crying.

"I can afford $800 a month," I said from the chair across from Louise. "Maybe I can see you once a month for that?" This would stretch our budget to the breaking point, but we'd make it for a while until I convinced the post office or some other non-screen-oriented place to hire me. Landscaping, maybe? One of those people who holds the stop sign in construction zones?

"No," Dr. Tanner said, shaking his head.

"Once every other month?" I asked. I had guessed at what he charged out of pocket based on what I'd paid other doctors. "How much do you charge out of pocket?"

"No insurance company is going to dictate how I treat my patients. You will come here as often as you need to for as long as you need to. For free."

For so long, I'd surrounded myself with volatile landscapes, volatile men, put myself in volatile situations. And then there was Mike, with his calm, steady, we're-in-it-together, and then this doctor, who had no reason to care but clearly did. I couldn't figure out what to say. I wanted to refuse, to figure out a way to pull my own weight, to be as self-reliant as I'd always been in the face of disaster, but I knew it was over. That part of me was no longer useful. The dizziness, in the most arduous of ways, had spun me into a world of kindness.

YEAR THIRTEEN

CHAPTER NINETEEN

Dr. Tanner had just returned from a migraine conference. His eyes were bright in the dim room. "There's a new drug coming out," he explained. "A whole new class of drugs. CGRPs they're called. The first drugs made to treat migraine specifically. Might be your ticket."

Eventually, the drug hit the market in the form of a shot that lasted three months. I dragged my feet, afraid to try it, annoyed by my fear. I went about my days, wrecked by 6:00 p.m., exhausted by the war my body was fighting all day as I got up early, packed lunches, got the kids out the door, worked, wrote, taught, grocery shopped, made dinner, helped with homework, ran the boys to soccer and baseball practice. It wasn't lost on me that I could now do all those things, but it was a push. Every day a struggle, every evening a snarly dizziness mad that I'd ignored all its rules throughout the day.

Not wanting to take advantage, I saw Dr. Tanner twice a month. He continued to tweak my medicines, continued to administer the two shots that chased out the dizziness, continued to charge me zero dollars, continued to mention the new drug. A three-month shot is not something you can reverse. It's not something you can stop taking because the side effects are debilitating or because, instead of helping, it makes the dizziness worse. I tried to imagine a three-month period of time I could be useless. The summer, maybe? The boys were seven. They needed a functioning adult in the house. Maybe the summer after they graduated high school? I tried to imagine another eleven years, tried to tell myself I could live with the current level of day-to-day dizziness. A person can only juggle for so long. Eventually, everything in the air comes crashing down to the floor.

Dr. Tanner hired a PA, Diane. I often saw her. She didn't push, but on occasion, she'd make vague mention of some other unnamed, horribly messed up patient like me who was having great luck with the new drug.

The price tag on the three-month shot was $540, and because it was a new drug, although FDA approved, no insurance companies were covering it, mine included. Because I was in the super messed up category, the recommended dose was two shots a month. So that was my excuse for a while. I didn't want to deliver pizzas.

But, in the way of big money corporate games, the company who manufactured the drug offered to give anyone who wanted to try it two months' worth of doses for free.

On a cold January morning, once the boys were off to school, I sat on the edge of my bed, the two shots and all the instructions spread out in front of me. My heart beat hard in my chest, as if a bear was clacking its teeth at me, angling up to charge.

I took a deep breath and watched the ceiling above slide to the left in my vision. Roxy Lou curled up on the carpet at my feet. "Alright," I said to her. "Alright. Here goes."

I injected myself once in each thigh. I lay back on the pillows and watched the sky out the window, waiting for something horrible to start happening. Three months of projectile vomiting? Three months of blindness? Three months of dizziness so bad I'd have to quit my jobs and hire a full-time nanny who accepted credit card payments?

The bright blue mass of Colorado sky outside jerked hard to the left and then slowly tracked back to the right and then jerked again and then miraculously stilled. I sat up. The walls and floors held still. The dog wasn't sloshing around on the carpet. I got up carefully, walked down the center of the hallway, able to keep track of where the walls were without running a finger along them. I stepped outside in my bare feet. The cold pavement stung my feet as I took a few steps. I was still on a boat, but we had found a calm bay. I walked out into the middle of the neighborhood road. As far as I could see, it stretched out and mostly held still. The parked cars along its edges remained firm and solid. I took off at a sprint, just to feel the freedom of it.

For weeks, I walked around in a daze, staring at one thing, then the next, as if I'd been thawed out from the Neanderthal days. I curled up against my boys, trying to make up for lost time. I stayed up late, I drank whiskey out of the bottle (once), I laughed and moved my head around freely.

I pushed it too far, of course. The dizziness came raging back if I got out of line, but that line had been moved far enough back that I had room to reconstruct myself.

YEAR SIXTEEN

CHAPTER TWENTY

Eight years into our working relationship, I asked Dr. Tanner, "Do you think this is as good as I'm ever going to get?"

The world still shifted and moved underneath me when I was working, when I was parenting, when I was trying so hard to be myself. No more Bering Sea winter water, but the Inside Passage was easily kicked up if I got up early, went to bed late, when the kids got into a screaming match, or when life delivered one of them a painful injustice, when work stressed me out, when there was too much sun or a storm rolled in, when I drank alcohol, when a room had the wrong kind of lights, when I got stuck with too many people for too long, and sometimes for no apparent reason at all. There were also short periods of time when the dizziness was so minimal, I could almost forget it was there.

Dr. Tanner breathed out a sigh at my question, regarded me from his seat against the wall. I wanted to be cured. We both know there is no cure for migraine.

"I don't know how much better you'll get," he said. "But we'll keep thinking widely, continue to make changes, support the ups and downs as best we can." He smiled easily, said, "We'll just keep working on it." And for the time being, that two-letter word that has pulled me from the depths time and time again was enough to keep my head above water.

■ ■ ■

The next day, a Saturday, Mike was at the firehouse, and I was doing endless loads of laundry. The boys were playing a video game, a jumble of long, gangly limbs on the couch downstairs. They had one week left of fifth grade, and both the soccer season and the spring hockey season had come to an end, which had granted us a weekend without any practices or games. I crouched down next to the arm of the couch. "You guys know I love you, right?"

"Yes, Mama," they both answered, rolling their eyes and throwing elbows at the interruption and the squishy question.

"You know I try really hard to fight through the dizziness but sometimes it gets me anyway, right?"

Nate set his controller down and looked at me. His smooth, boyish face had started to take on the look of the man he will become. "It's okay, Mama," he said with enough empathy to make me think he would save the whole world one day. "Really."

"It's not always okay. I'd probably be less moody if I was a healthy person. Have more patience and more energy," I said. "You know, be more fun."

Wes set his controller down too. The video game continued on in the background.

"Life's not perfect, Mama." Wes laid his hand in the crook of my elbow with that same spark of we've-got-this-anyway in his eye that used to light up my dad's face. "And we still have fun."

CODA

This was to be a book about living in the kingdom of the sick, but it recently made the turn to restitution narrative. I found my way out of jail. I've been free of the constant dizziness for close to two years. I am learning the world again, learning myself again, taking tentative steps toward trusting that I get to stay in the kingdom of the well. Migraine is a personal demon. No two are the same. Every migraineur knows that what works for their migraine afflicted friend may or may not work for them.

In year seventeen of the chronic dizziness, I got COVID, and everything stopped working: the delicate combination of drugs that took the edge off, my mind, my body, my ability to push through it all. Diane and Dr. Tanner began seeing me together to try to figure out next steps, to try to haul me back to where I'd been, but I'd turned to water and was spilling out on the floor, evaporating into nothing.

How could this story possibly get worse? you might be thinking, and I was too.

We all decided more cooks in the kitchen wasn't a bad idea, so I took what Mike and I had scraped together into a savings account and began flinging myself all over the country, putting myself in front of anyone who specialized in severe, hard to treat, chronic migraine. I ran headfirst into several dead ends, and then I landed at the Migraine and Neuro Rehab Center run by Dr. Kyle Bills, a PhD neuroscientist in Utah.

It started with a phone call. Mike, the boys, and I were driving back home from visiting family across the country. I had filled out the I-want-to-be-a-patient fields on Dr. Bills's website, and unexpectedly, he called me himself.

"Do your symptoms get worse throughout the day?"

"Yes."

"Is it worse when you get hungry?"

"Yes."

"Does your brain feel slower than usual?"

"Yes."

After ten minutes of Dr. Bills asking questions that were 100 percent relevant and that 100 percent described my daily life, like some sort of scientific fortune teller sprung out of the ether, I said, "It feels like you've known me forever."

Mike threw me a look from the driver's seat. It was his *now's not the time to act weird* look. His *everything's riding on this* look.

Dr. Bills went on to explain that he was finishing up a study investigating the theory that glucose levels affect migraine, which was based on research begun at Johns Hopkins Hospital in 1936.

In that study, one thousand children with myoclonic epilepsy were treated with a ketogenic diet, which stabilizes glucose levels in the body. The results showed 54 percent were freed from seizures, and an additional 26 percent showed marked improvement. Research shows that epilepsy and migraine share similar underlying mechanisms, such as hyperexcitability in the brain. Dr. Bills set out to see if what worked for epilepsy might work for migraine and to further explore and better understand the metabolic component of migraine.

Dr. Bills sent me to LabCorps close to home for a three-hour glucose tolerance test. "You're not going to like me very much after this," he said.

My fasting glucose was in the normal range, as it had been in every other blood work I'd done, but when I drank the disgusting sugary liquid, my glucose plummeted rather than rose, and the dizziness and headache and brain fog raged unhindered. I found a chair in the lobby of the hospital outside LabCorps, curled up, and lay there, willing the room still for hours until I could drive home.

Typically, when you eat carbs or sugar, it's broken down into glucose, causing your blood glucose level to rise. Your body then produces insulin, dumps it into the bloodstream to move the glucose to the cells to be used for energy or stored for later. In lay terms, ingesting sugar should not make your blood glucose level drop, it should make it rise.

Dr. Bills works with people remotely, but I felt the need to set eyes on him, to decide if he was a snake oil salesman or the real deal before I submitted myself to a ketogenic diet. I'd tried the Heal Your Headache diet, had bought Alicia Wolf's *The Dizzy Cook*, had been religious about it all for months, years at a time. So far, changing my diet had been an enormous effort for minimal results. I wanted to believe Dr. Bills was on to something, but it was hard to muster the energy necessary to overhaul my diet once again.

I suffered the flight to Salt Lake City, the drive to Provo, slept fourteen hours in a glorious hotel bed, and showed up to Dr. Bills's clinic the next morning, worn thin and completely blown out. We sat in his office with big windows and a bigger desk. He's about my age, but everywhere I am calloused and moody, he is sunshine.

He showed me my three-hour glucose test compared to others in his study. A graph of the afflicted that my numbers matched. "Wait," I said. "There's a whole slew of other people who feel the same as me?"

"Yep." He nodded and went on to explain his understanding of the science behind the numbers, the metabolic mechanisms that had gone haywire deep inside my brain, and the ways he'd found to calm everything down that worked for most of the folks involved in his study. He sat back, gave me the time I needed to assimilate what he was saying, which my brain could only sort of do, and ask all the questions I had, of which there were about a million.

He explained the science behind why leveling off my blood glucose level would lead my brain into the calm space that had eluded it for so long. He took a deep breath at one point, a pause, as I readjusted in the chair, trying to get the thirty-foot seas that were tossing me about to ease up.

"Eighteen years is an extraordinary amount of time," he said, watching me closely.

The weight of it, the sincerity. I was not an illness to be dealt with in a ten-minute window of time. I was a person whose whole life had been swallowed up by this.

"Yeah." My voice cracked on the rocks of the truth. I blinked at the gathering tears, afraid to hope that this just might be the thing to set me free.

Dr. Bills tilted his head. "My mom suffered with migraine the whole time I was growing up."

I fell still in the chair. My heart seized up, thinking of Wes and Nate.

"I get how tough it is. It was hard on her."

"What about for you?" I whisper asked.

"I just wanted to find a way to help her."

"So you went and got a PhD to study migraine?"

"Yep." He laughed, sunny disposition shining everywhere. Not a snake oil salesman. Another man like Dr. Tanner, willing to get into the middle of it with patients, to stomp around in the mucky corners with no concern for keeping his shoes clean.

Before I left that day, Dr. Bills had me take a neurocognitive test. My scores were consistent with someone with a traumatic brain injury. I was stunned. I knew this, of course, that my brain felt like mud, that I was exerting way more energy than normal to try to make it work.

"Don't worry," Dr. Bills said based on whatever my face was doing when he delivered the news. "You'll take the test again after three months of keto, and you'll see a huge difference. Back to normal functioning, I would guess." Which sounded a little snaky, but I would see for myself, already knowing that I would follow his protocol based on the science, but also based on the trust he'd built between us, knowingly or not.

Next step, Dr. Bills fitted me with a ten-day continuous glucose monitor to get some baseline data, with me eating as I typically did. Back home, each morning, my glucose level would be in the normal range of 70 to 100 mg/dL. But after eating, I regularly recorded glucose readings in the forties and fifties. The constant alarming of the glucose monitor became the background of our lives.

Mike lost his mind. On the ambulance, they jump into action if someone drops below 60 mg/dL. They have the patient who is typically weak, shaky, having a hard time thinking, maybe has a headache or feels dizzy, eat or drink something sugary to pull their blood glucose levels back up to the more normal 70 to 100 range. But in my case, anything sugary drove my blood glucose even lower. He hated that the fix he'd been taught wouldn't work. That we just had to wait out the low numbers.

I found it revelatory. My symptoms followed the numbers. The lower they got, the worse the dizziness raged, the louder and more insistent the alarm became. My internal made external. Finally. No more convincing, no more wondering if I was overdramatizing, making it all up. An alarm screaming over and over for all to hear: THIS IS NOT RIGHT.

Once in those ten days, while driving and talking to Mike on the phone over the hands-free business in the car, my blood glucose dropped into the thirties.

"Pull over!" Mike yelled into the phone over the sound of my monitor alarming.

"I'm fine," I insisted, ignoring the cars jerking into my lane because they actually weren't. "I feel like this at least once a week." To be chronically ill is to normalize all sorts of abnormal things in order to get by. If you spend too much time focused on how difficult everything is, you've got no energy left for parenting, for wife-ing, working, for any sort of original thought. So you tell yourself cars jumping around in lanes is just that, nothing more, and you get on with your day.

In addition to the lows, the continuous glucose monitor showed that rather than the typical two-hour time frame for levels to return to the premeal level after eating, mine would drop and rise and get back to where I started in thirty to sixty minutes, depending on what I ate.

Every night, I stared at the graph tracking my blood glucose for the day. I felt like a kid who'd aced a test. Except that I was earning a failing grade and that was the best news ever. All the times doctors had bustled into the room to report with a smile that my lab results, MRI, CT scans were "Fantastic! All normal!" I needed to fail a test to engage them, to get them to believe me, and here, finally, I had what the medical system had been demanding for so long. Hard data to prove I wasn't making it all up. Not just words but numbers. I understood that this is what I'd been fighting for so long. This, along with the dizziness, was the root of the exhaustion. The vast majority of clinicians I'd seen devalued words over numbers. They let numbers on tests wash away the words of the story I was trying to tell. It was rarely a question of having run the wrong test. Typically, it was a question of whether to believe me when the words didn't line up with the numbers on the test results in front of them.

I wanted to print out the continuous glucose monitor graph and post it on the fridge, get it printed onto a T-shirt and wear it around every day. Print it out and mail it to every doctor I'd seen across the hailstorm of the last eighteen years.

Reactive hypoglycemia, sometimes called postprandial hypoglycemia, is the name of the condition in which blood sugar drops in response to ingesting carbohydrates. My understanding of Dr. Bills's theory is that the hyperactivity in the hypothalamus, due to either the quick changes in glucose levels and/or the reactive hypoglycemia, agitates the nervous system and triggers migraine in those susceptible to migraine.

Over the past two decades, I had identified and done my best to avoid or preemptively address all the triggers the world contained—noise, lights, sun, storms, alcohol, chocolate, bad sleep, stress—all the while eating breakfast, lunch, and dinner, which were the biggest triggers of all. I should take a moment here and say I wasn't eating cake and cookies and chips all day long. The Heal Your Headache diet had led me to notice I felt worse when I ate gluten, so I was avoiding it at this point. And big loads of sugar never made me feel very good. I was eating oatmeal and green smoothies, lots of fruit and veggies, rice and stir-fries, salads with a delicious honey mustard dressing I'd discovered.

Next step, ketosis for three months.

I'd never paid attention to carbs in food. Turns out oatmeal, rice, fruit, carrots even, have a lot of carbs. Not to mention how many store-bought items sugar is added to. "Fifteen grams of carbs a day," Dr. Bills said, "tops." And lots of fat. Heavy whipping cream in my coffee, full fat yogurt. I'd spent a lifetime vaguely afflicted by the idea that fat was bad. Not so in ketosis.

Within twenty-four hours of ketosis, things began to soften, to settle. Some tight, invisible fist inside my chest flexed its fingers for the first time in almost two decades, and I took a full breath.

Back in our hunter gatherer days, human bodies had two modes of processing food for energy. Two factories, let's say. The glucose factory ran in the summer, when there were fruits and veggies to harvest. The ketosis factory kicked to life in the winter, when the glucose foods ran out and our ancestors ate mastodons or whatever other animals they could catch, reducing their diet to fat and protein.

The year-round abundance of fruits and vegetables in our lives now, not to mention all the processed food, keep us in the glucose, so the ketosis factory in our bodies these days remains closed. But in a pinch, or because Dr. Bills tells us to, if there's not enough glucose to burn for energy, our bodies will kick the dust off and start up the ketosis factory that burns fat rather than glucose for energy. By eating only fifteen grams of carbs a day, I forced the shutdown of the glucose factory and the start-up of the ketosis factory for the first time ever in my body. This did not feel good. The keto flu, it's often called. Dr. Bills called from his car on his drive home to remind me it would pass after a few days and not to give up.

Within two weeks, the brain fog cleared out. Completely. Along with all of the dizziness. I stared at the world slack-jawed from this new place of stillness and with a clear mind. How amazing to be able to land on words without a struggle, to stay up after dark, to go to the boys' orchestra concerts, to curl into Mike and sip whiskey to no ill effects except the normal ones.

I wanted a do-over on every important thing. I asked Mike if we could get married again, I asked the boys if we could go down the swirly slides together at the nearby park, where they would beg to do so when toddlers and every time I'd had to say no because swirly slides are not for dizzy people.

Wes, thirteen at the time, said, "Ahhh, maybe. If it's dark out."

Mike said, "Do you think you're going to talk this much from now on?"

To wake up without misery, to drive at night, listening to music turned up, to take the dogs for a walk, to discuss the missing middle school assignments, to work, to simply exist in the kingdom of the well, is bliss.

In those early weeks, I was afraid it wouldn't last. I was afraid I had a short window of freedom. I wanted the four of us to quit our lives, become surf bums in Costa Rica. Nate said, "Ummm, I think I need to stay in school." To which I replied, a little too wild-eyed, "School's for fools!"

Nate, Wes, and Mike watched me carefully out of the corners of their eyes. Nate and Wes had only known me sick. Mike and I had been friends before the dizziness, but he had only ever been in a relationship with the sick version of me. The free version of me was overwhelming us all.

"How about we sell the house, buy a van, and live out of it with both dogs and the kids!?? It'll be amazing!!"

Mike patted my knee.

At the one-month mark, I spent hours, whole days, curled up on the couch on the back deck, watching the late summer trees, trying to process everything that had happened. To emerge back into the world after eighteen years in jail is to have sensitive skin.

I watched the tree branches against the forever blue of the Colorado sky and thought about how perilously close I'd come to ending my own life. Doctoring is a hard business, and so is Patienting. The medical system so often remains hyperfocused on our physical symptoms. But after a long time of physical suffering, the emotional symptoms tangle up with the physical, like balloon strings subjected to a strong wind.

The clinicians who encouraged a few steps back from that ledge of suicide were the ones who didn't ignore the vast emotional toll the illness was taking. What I needed more than anything was for both sides of the struggle to be equally recognized within the same space. The clinicians, like Dr. Tanner, who made room for both, who let me talk, who let me ask the darker questions, were the true healers. It doesn't matter that Dr. Tanner wasn't the one who landed on the solution in the end, he's the one who saved my life.

■ ■ ■

I think a lot about hope and why I never gave up. I hate hope. It smells like mayonnaise gone bad. And yet I never quite shed it. In the January before my dad died, I had driven the family car a long way one afternoon, ignoring the check engine light, which was begging me to notice that all the coolant had leaked out. I melted the engine block. My punishment was that I had to rebuild it, starting at 7:00 a.m. every weekend morning for months under my dad's close supervision. I had no idea how to rebuild an engine. All I knew was that my dad was pissed and it was going to suck.

He rebuilt engines all the time. It seemed much more straight-forward for him to do the work.

I was given an incredibly low budget and a list of parts I had to round up on my own by going around to the various junkyards in rural Tennessee, most of which were populated by vicious, slobbery junkyard dogs and a sketchy man in overalls.

My dad would smoke and drink his coffee, perched on a stool he'd dragged out to the driveway on those early mornings we spent rebuilding, and point out tools and where to use them and shake his head when I scraped half my knuckles off.

We were both annoyed at the whole situation at first, but eventually, I got interested in understanding what connects to what and how the whole of it worked. He left his perch on the stool and leaned under the hood with me, explaining it all, nodded at how I learned to move in the tight spaces, smiled when I picked up the right tool before he had to tell me. A parting gift in a way. A basic knowledge of car engines and how to work on them that would save me thousands of dollars I didn't have as the long series of old cars I would drive across the next decade would break down on roadsides all over the country.

In his squinty, hard-to-read way, he used those early mornings to build on what he'd been talking about on that slow drive back from Florida and had been showing me through his own significant struggle with life all along. That the physicality of life is uncomfortable, and that's okay. That life will toss you into impossible emotional landscapes, and that's okay too, because at the very center of him and me, and most all of us, lies a slow, heavy ballast of resilience. It just takes a lot of life beating you up, of life demanding a lot from you, to land on its shores, to recognize how wide and solid it is.

The cold rain of Alaska, the terrifying Cessna rides among mountains hidden in fog, all the times I came face to face with bears, the shipwreck, the waterspout strong enough to sink the boat and leave me adrift, along with the way my dad was forced to live so often right on the edge of everything coming apart— they all reinforced that underneath the fear and lack of control is that reservoir of resilience you can count on. Knowing this calmed me in the time I needed it most, allowed me to define myself in a specific way in that slippery sloped kingdom of the sick, allowed me to find enough hope to not give up through all the doctors and dead ends and horrible days, even though hope and I will forever have a contentious relationship.

For all the times I've obsessed and worried over the way my illness has shaped Wes and Nate's lives, for all the peanut butter and jelly sandwiches they made themselves for dinner when Mike was at work and I could not get myself off the couch, I am starting to see glimmers that what my dad passed to me has passed to them too. A ballast they will need for their own lives. I watch them from the corners, which is where they prefer I hang out now that they are fourteen. They are gathering themselves for their own journeys, pulling away from me, as they need to. Me being ill for the first twelve years of their lives hasn't been easy for them, and I would venture to say it's mostly been hard, but for better or for worse, through it all, they have forged their own reservoirs of resilience.

It terrifies me to think I got so lost in illness that I almost let them go. Every day that I get to see them do all the normal things—bicker with each other, spend too much time staring at their phones, moan dramatically when asked to mow the lawn—I say a silent thank you, to the universe, to my dad, to myself, to the clinicians who are good at the harder parts of their jobs, that I am around for it.

We are too busy right now with the daily concerns of raising two teens, working, keeping the dogs off the furniture, staying on top of the never-ending laundry, and figuring out what the kids will eat that still constitutes healthy, but I will get Mike to marry me again. This time, I imagine we will elope. On a beach somewhere at dusk, holding his hands, just before the officiant says, *You may now kiss the bride*, I will find a way to tell him that his love, steady and whole from the beginning, and forged as it has been through hardship, is and always has been the framework within which I want to live forever.

Dr. Bills's protocol calls for a slow increase of carbs after the initial three months of keto to find your own threshold where migraine symptoms return. My threshold is pretty low. No more ketosis, but I still eat a very low carb diet, every once in a while collecting my Mama Tax on one of the boys' ice cream cones, knowing that a couple bites will cause the dizziness to gather itself for an hour or so somewhere deep inside my head. In a weird way, I kind of like it. It's like a visit from an old enemy, now with stringy, gray hair and bony arms, but the eyes are just as scary as ever. A reminder of how desperate life can get and how not-desperate my life currently is. I can still get dizzy, irritable, want everything quiet and dimly lit when big storms roll in, when I feel stressed, when I don't sleep well, but a couple Advil clear it all out now.

The new receptionist at Dr. Tanner's clinic doesn't know me. She was probably in fifth grade when I first dragged myself into those dimly lit rooms, in middle and high school across the years when everyone would give the toddler, and then the preschool, and then the elementary school versions of Nate and Wes knuckles on our way back to the treatment room. I love that I go so rarely now that she's got to look on the schedule to recall my name.

Dr. Tanner and the PA who took over Diane's job still cook in my migraine kitchen. A CGRP along with every-three-month Botox add enough stability that I can tolerate a few extra carbs a day. My MTWTFSS holder is remarkably empty. Life in all its possibilities spreads out before me, wide and open as the sky seventy-five feet up in the evergreens of Missoula.

Dr. Bills will seek publication of his study involving three hundred chronic migraineurs like me in the fall of 2025 or spring of 2026. I'm not at liberty to discuss his findings before they are published, but I can say I'm not a singular case study. There are a lot of other former chronic migraineurs out there, sitting on their back decks, reveling in a whole new life.

■ ■ ■

That summer I tried to save the old growth for the murrelets, it didn't work. Our boss never sent Glen to a class, which left me the only certified climber on our district. According to Forest Service regulations, a minimum of two climbers is necessary in case one gets in trouble and needs rescue, so I couldn't climb to check for murrelet nests.

One morning, I got up hours before daybreak and drove one of the Forest Service work trucks to an old growth stand on a steep hillside in the middle of the uninhabited island where I'd spent the week searching for goshawks. It was overcast, rain misting the mossy forest floor and the thick trunks of trees. Still preoccupied with murrelets, I wanted to see for myself if they were using this particular old growth stand to bed down at night, deep in the middle of the island.

I parked at the edge of the vast swath of trees too big to put my arms around, left the hood of my raincoat off, and walked the dirt road in the pitch black of the early morning until the first orangey-gray of morning lit up the wispy clouds tangled in the branches of the canopy high overhead.

The first two murrelets dropped from a branch above, their impossibly small, stout bodies falling fast to the ground until the frantic beating of too-short wings caught and lifted them in surprising, spiraling arcs as they followed the corridor of the dimly lit road toward the shore, twenty-seven miles away. My heart crushed at the idea that this is what it had come to for them. Before humans came in and took all the good timber from the shores, they didn't have to travel so far to find an old growth stand. It seemed hard to believe that traveling such great distances every day was sustainable.

As color washed into the sky, more murrelets woke up. They continued to drop all around me, two at a time, from their bedded down branches high above, their bodies all wrong, it seemed, for how far they had to go.

I had expected to see ten, maybe twenty, murrelets that morning, but they kept coming. Hundreds swooped and spiraled past on either side of my body, making me hold my breath. They crowded the sky overhead, spiraling in and out of each other, more adept at flying than I had ever given them credit for. It was a death drop at first, but it seemed once they got going, they were fine. They called and swooped and dove, every single one wing to wing in perfect symphony with their partners, breaking open the silence of the morning like a sparkling geode in the biggest demonstration of We I'd ever seen in the face of a long distance to travel.

ABOUT THE AUTHOR

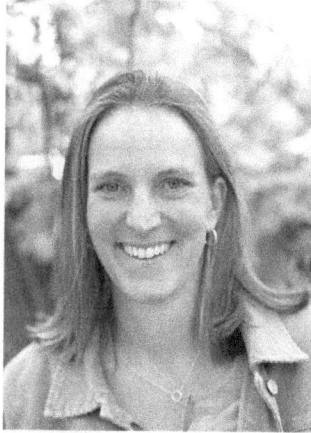

Photo credit: Ben Klaus

Rachel Weaver is a writer of fiction and nonfiction. Her debut novel, *Point of Direction*, was chosen by the ABA in spring 2014 as a Top Ten Debut and awarded the 2015 Willa Cather Award for Contemporary Fiction. Her second novel, The Last Run, is due out in June 2026. Prior to earning her MFA in writing and poetics from Naropa University, Weaver worked for the Forest Service in Alaska studying bears, raptors, and songbirds. She is on faculty at Wilkes University's low-residency MFA program and at Lighthouse Writers Workshop. She lives in Colorado.